International Migration and Wellness Innovation in the United States, Sweden, and Japan

Edited by Kazumi Hoshino

Kazumi Hoshino, Winston Tseng,
Nancy Hikoyeda and Dolores Gallagher-Thompson

KAZAMA SHOBO

Table of Contents

Acknowledgments   1

Introduction   5

Part 1 International Migration and Wellness Innovation in the United States and Sweden

Chapter 1 Cultural Identity and Intergenerational Relationships among   17
Chinese, Japanese, and Peruvian Americans
Kazumi Hoshino, Winston Tseng, Nancy Hikoyeda, & Dolores
Gallagher-Thompson

Chapter 2 Cultural Identity and Intergenerational Support among   41
Asian and Hispanic Americans in the United States
Kazumi Hoshino, Winston Tseng, Nancy Hikoyeda, & Dolores
Gallagher-Thompson

Chapter 3 Cultural Identity, Intergenerational Relationships, and Social   65
Policies among Diverse Immigrants in Sweden
Kazumi Hoshino

Part 2 International Migration and Wellness Innovation in Japan

Chapter 4 Development of the Multigroup Ethnic Identity Measure-   81
Revised Japanese Version
Kazumi Hoshino

Chapter 5 Ethnic Identity, Intergenerational Support, and Psychosocial   109
Development among Younger and Older Adults in Japan
Kazumi Hoshino

Part 3 Future Directions

Chapter 6 International Migration, Wellness, and Social Policies in the   141
United States, Sweden, and Japan
Kazumi Hoshino

Chapter 7 Conclusions   163
Kazumi Hoshino

Appendix   175

Appendix 1 Informed Consent Form of Cultural Identity and
Intergenerational Relationships among Diverse Adults in the United States
(Chapters 1 and 2)

Appendix 2 Demographic Form of Cultural Identity and Intergenerational

Relationships (Chapters 1 and 2)

Appendix 3 Interview Protocol of Cultural Identity and Intergenerational
Relationships (Chapters 1 and 2)

Appendix 4 The Multigroup Ethnic Identity Measure-Revised (Chapter 4)

Appendix 5 The Multigroup Ethnic Identity Measure-Revised Japanese
Version (Chapter 4)

Contributor Biographies 189

Acknowledgments

Kazumi Hoshino

This book is based on several research projects in the United States, Sweden, and Japan (each Principal Investigator: Kazumi Hoshino). The author was a Visiting Scholar at the School of Public Health (04/2010-09/2011) as well as the Institute of Personality and Social Research (10/2012-03/2013) at the University of California at Berkeley. The author was also granted a Residential Faculty Fellowship Award by the Institute of East Asian Studies and served as a Residential Faculty Fellow (10/2011-09/2012). The University of California at Berkeley has demonstrated diversity as one of their official missions. The University of California at Berkeley has emphasized diversity and has aimed that each individual, who reflects gender, age, education, socioeconomic status, culture, ethnicity, religion, and sexual orientation, is equally respected. In particular, the University has enlightened others by supporting minorities from their perspectives.

The author wishes to thank my Faculty Sponsors, Dr. S. Leonard Syme and Dr. Winston Tseng for inviting me to the School of Public Health at the University of California at Berkeley. The author also acknowledges that Dr. Andrew E. Scharlach had supported me as my Mentor during the term. We conducted the International Symposium on Healthy Aging at the University of California at Berkeley in 2010. Dr. Andrew E. Scharlach and the author edited our book entitled Healthy Aging in Sociocultural Context (published by Routledge) with the contributors, including Dr. Winston Tseng as well as American, Swedish, and Japanese professors. We also published the Japanese Version entitled Kenko Choju no Shakai Bunkateki Bunmyaku from Kazamashobo Press.

After the author was a Visiting Scholar to the Department of Human Development and Family Studies at the Pennsylvania State University (04/2013-03/2014), the author invited Dr. Winston Tseng to the International Symposium in Japan in 2014 and the 2015 UC Berkeley International Symposium at Osaka University. Dr. Winston Tseng and the author examined cultural identity, intergenerational relationships, and mental health in the United States, Sweden, and Japan in the 2014 conference. The 2015 International Symposium enlightened wellness innovation from the viewpoint of translational research in natural sciences and social sciences in the United States, China, and Japan. The author also invited Dr. Linda Neuhauser to the International Symposium in Japan in 2016, which endorsed multicultural health care for immigrants in the United States, Germany, Sweden, China, and Japan. The author is proud of our important collaboration with the University of California at Berkeley.

The author appreciates that Global Collaboration Center and Osaka School of International Public Policy at Osaka University invited me as a Visiting Professor. The author also acknowledges each sponsorship of the international symposium and the international seminar at Osaka University: Global Collaboration Center; Division of Public Health at the Graduate School of Medicine; and Center for International Affairs at the Graduate School of Science. Finally, the author wishes to thank President of Kazamashobo Press, Ms. Keiko Kazama for allowing me to publish this innovative book, in which Grant-In-Aid for Scientific Research (16HP5171) was granted the author by the Japan Society for Promotion of Science.

In this book, most chapters were presented at the following conferences and were written with the author's expanded data analyses and deepened conclusions. In addition, Chapter 4 was first printed on the Central Japanese Journal of Psychology, and Figure 7-1 as well as Table 7-1 of Chapter 7 was formerly presented on the Compilation and Documentation on Refugees and Migrants Quarterly. The author appreciates these scientific journals for their agreements with reprinting the paper, the figure, and the table for this publication. Furthermore, the author would like to express sincere gratitude to the research grants by the academic associations, which have recognized excellence of the international research projects.

Chapter 1: Hoshino, K., Tseng, W., Hikoyeda, N., Gallagher-Thompson, D., Ventura, J., & Inoue, H. (2012). Poster presented at the 65th Annual Scientific Meeting of the Gerontological Society of America in San Diego (funded by the Foundation of Japanese Certification Board for Clinical Psychologists).

Chapter 2: Tseng, W., Hoshino, K., Hikoyeda, N., Gallagher-Thompson, D., Ventura, J., & Inoue, H. (2012). Poster presented at the 65th Annual Scientific Meeting of the Gerontological Society of America in San Diego (funded by the Foundation of Japanese Certification Board for Clinical Psychologists).

Chapter 3: Hoshino, K. (2014). Paper presented at the 78th Annual Convention of the Japanese Psychological Association in Kyoto (funded by the Health Science Center).

Chapter 4: Hoshino, K., & Zarit, S.H. (2014). Development of the Multigroup Ethnic Identity Measure-Revised Japanese Version, *Central Japanese (Tokai) Journal of Psychology, 8*, 28-39 (funded by the Japan Society for Promotion of Science).

4

Chapter 5: Hoshino, K., Zarit, S.H. et al. (2011). Poster presented at the 64th Annual Scientific Meeting of the Gerontological Society of America in New Orleans (funded by the Japan Society for Promotion of Science).

Chapter 6: Hoshino, K. (2012). Paper presented at the Residential Faculty Fellowship Awardee Seminar in Berkeley (funded by the Residential Faculty Fellowship Award of the Institute of East Asian Studies at the University of California at Berkeley).

Chapter 7: Hoshino, K. (2016). Multidisciplinary and Multicultural Support Model for Immigrants on Legal Issues, *Compilation and Documentation on Refugees and Migrants Quarterly* (in press) (funded by the Association of Japanese Clinical Psychology).

Introduction

Kazumi Hoshino

International Migration, Cultural Identity, and Intergenerational Relationships

Dramatic demographic changes have occurred over the past few decades in the United States, Sweden, as well as Japan, and minority populations have transcended the number of European Americans since 2011 in the United States (U.S. Census, 2014). Although the majority of minorities were Hispanic Americans and Asian Americans, previous family studies seldom differentiated how specific cohort, immigrant generation, and ethnicity affect cultural identity and intergenerational relationships among underrepresented ethnic groups. Of those, commonalities of migration aims among Hispanic Americans and Asian Americans are to obtain better opportunities for education, careers, freedom, and individualism. Researchers can see this trend by reflecting on each political system, economic instability, and familism norms of the migrating individuals (Cheng, Li, Leung, & Chan, 2011; Crivello, 2011; Dong, Chang, Wong, & Simon, 2012; Leinaweaver, 2010; Iwamasa, & Iwasaki, 2011).

Worldwide geographic mobility has shaped transnationality and has influenced cultural identity and intergenerational relationships. The current challenges in the United States, Sweden, and Japan are how each generation can promote lifespan development mutually in the midst of considerable family diversity (Fingerman, Miller, Birditt, & Zarit, 2009;

Kim, Zarit, Eggebeen, Birditt, & Fingerman, 2011; Fingerman, VanderDrift, Dotterer, Birditt, & Zarit, 2011), and how they can actualize social integration in unprecedented multicultural and multigenerational communities (Hoshino, 2012). Reflecting the importance of socioeconomic status, international students, migrant workers, and immigrants are more vulnerable to societal, social, and familial changes than native-born nationals.

Definition and Dimensions of Wellness

According to Berkeley Wellness.com, wellness is optimal physical, mental and emotional well-being, a preventive way of living that reduces --sometimes even eliminates-- the need for remedies. It emphasizes personal responsibility for making the lifestyle choices and self-care decisions that will improve the quality of your life (Berkeley Wellness.com, 2015). Wellness transcends the concept of health, which is defined as a state of complete physical, mental, and social well-being, and not merely the absence of diseases (WHO, 2015), and refers to multidimensional perspectives of health. In other words, wellness is a conscious, self-directed and evolving process of achieving full potential (National Institute, 2015) and is a dynamic process of changes and human lifespan development (SHCS, UC Davis, 2015).

Substance Abuse and Mental Health Services Administration (SAMHSA) at the National Institute of Mental Health has implemented SAMHSA Wellness Initiatives to raise awareness of health disparities between people with serious mental and/or substance use disorders and the general population in the United States (SAMHSA, 2015). Wellness consists of eight dimensions: emotional, social, environmental, financial, intellectual, occupational, physical, and spiritual (Smarbrick, 2006). Learning about the

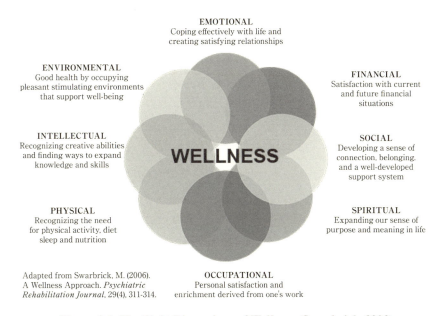

Figure 0-1. The Eight Dimensions of Wellness (Smarbrick, 2006)

eight dimensions of wellness will help people choose how to pursue wellness in their daily lives.

Wellness Innovation at the University of California at Berkeley

The School of Public Health at the University of California at Berkeley has published the UC Berkeley Wellness Letter since 1984 (SPH, UCB, 2015). Dr. S. Leonard Syme developed the Berkeley Wellness Guide to promote physical and mental health and to reduce barriers to access health care services among Asian immigrants in the San Francisco Bay Area in 1986. Tseng & Neuhauser (2015) implemented China Migrant Worker Wellness Project to improve health disparities among migrant workers in China and conducted intervention to solve problems of physical and mental health, and family relationships among migrant youth and adults. Reflecting such innovative community-based initiatives, the University of California established UC Living Well Wellness Initiatives to encourage campus community members to live healthier lifestyles since 2007 (UCR, 2015). The main strategic goals are to improve health and quality of life, and to build cultures of wellness that support healthy lifestyles in members.

In addition, the Tang Center at the University of California at Berkeley provides comprehensive medical services and comprehensive counseling services, including individual, group, and career counseling (UHS, 2015). Faculty and staff can use the occupational health clinic, career counseling／workshops, wellness programs, rehabilitation, and other counseling services. The staff believe that health is multidimensional: Physical, mental, environmental, emotional, social, and spiritual. The Center embraces working collaboratively with clients, campus, and local providers using the strengths of a multidisciplinary approach. Thus, the Tang Center strengthens diversity and encourages wellness innovation.

Outline of This Book

The author will shed light on how international migration has interacted with wellness, in particular the important dimensions: emotional and social. The emotional dimension refers to coping effectively with life and creating satisfying relationships, while social dimension is defined as developing a sense of connection, belonging, and a well-developed support system. In this publication, the author will focus on cultural identity and intergenerational support and social policies of healthy aging among older adults in terms of social dimension. Emotional dimension will be analyzed from the perspectives of intergenerational relationships. It is essential to clarify how international migration may affect wellness among immigrants in the United States, Sweden, and Japan in terms of social dimension (i.e., cultural identity, intergenerational support, social policies of elderly health care and social services) and emotional dimension (i.e., intergenerational relationships), while immigrants may try to maintain consistency and face changes in their lives in the transitions from their home countries to their new countries.

This book consists of four parts. Part 1 will shed light on cultural identity, intergenerational relationships, and intergenerational support among Hispanic Americans and Asian Americans in the United States. This part will also enlighten cultural identity, intergenerational relationships, and social policies of mental health among diverse immigrants in Sweden. In chapter 1, based on the Cultural Identity Theory (Banks, 2006) and the Intergenerational Solidarity Theory (Bengtson, & Schrader, 1982; Bengtson, & Roberts, 1991; Roberts, & Bengtson, 1990; Roberts, & Bengtson, 1996; Silverstein, Gans, Rowenstein, Giarruso, & Bengtson, 2010), the authors will develop the Interview Protocol and will clarify commonalities and differences in cultural identity and intergenerational relationships from the viewpoint of Chinese, Japanese, and Peruvian Americans in their forties and fifties who have lived less than 30 years in the United States and have at least one child born in the United States. In chapter 2, the authors will examine associations between cultural identity and intergenerational support among children, adults, and elderly parents of Hispanic Americans and Asian Americans from the viewpoint of first generation adult immigrants in the United States. Chapter 3 will first focus on social policies of mental health and social inclusion in Sweden. Second, the author will examine mental health in terms of cultural identity and intergenerational support, and intergenerational relationships among immigrants to Sweden from Asia and South/East European countries as well as refugees from the Middle-East and Africa. Third, this chapter will clarify how these factors have affected mental health among diverse immigrants.

Part 2 will analyze associations between ethnic identity, intergenerational support, and psychosocial development among younger adults and older adults in Japan. In chapter 4, the author will develop the Multigroup Ethnic Identity Measure-Revised (Japanese Version) to evaluate ethnic identity of native born nationals as well as immigrants who use the Japanese language in Japan. The author will examine how ethnic identity may correlate to intergenerational support and psychosocial development among younger and older adults in Japan in chapter 5. Although Japan has been a homogeneous nation, consistency and/or inconsistency of ethnic identity among younger generations and older generations in relation to intergenerational support and psychosocial development may be emerging.

Part 3 will describe an international comparative study of social policies and healthy aging in the United States, Sweden, and Japan. Finally, the author will conclude associations between international migration and wellness in the three countries. In chapter 6, the author will view Chinese migration to the United States, Sweden, and Japan, and will conduct comparative research on social policies of elderly health care and social welfare in the three countries. The author will also identify how social policies may affect healthy aging among Chinese immigrants in the United States, Sweden, and Japan. Chapter 7 will demonstrate the associations between international migration and wellness from the perspectives of social dimension such as cultural identity, intergenerational support, and social policies of elderly care, as well as emotional dimension, including intergenerational relationships in the three countries.

REFERENCES

Banks, J. (1976). The emerging stages of ethnicity: Implications for staff development. *Educational Leadership, 34*(3), 190-193.

Banks, J. (2006). *Cultural diversity and education: Foundations, curriculum, and teaching (5 th ed.).* Boston: Pearson Education.

Bengtson, V.L., & Roberts, R.E.L. (1991). Intergenerational solidarity in aging families: An example of formal theory construction. *Journal of Marriage and Family, 53,* 856-870.

Bengtson, V.L., & Schrader, S.S. (1982). Parent-child relations. In D. Mangen & W. Peterson (Eds.) *Handbook of research instruments in social gerontology* (pp.115-185). Minneapolis: University of Minnesota Press.

Berkeley Wellness. com (2015). What is wellness? Retrieved July 12, 2015 from http://www.berkeleywellness.com/about-us

Cheng, S.-T., Li, K.-K., Leung, E.M.F., & Chan, A.C.M. (2011). Social exchanges and subjective well-being: Do sources of positive and negative exchanges matter? *The Journals of Gerontology Series B: Psychological Sciences and Social Sciences, 66B*(6), 708-718.

Crivello, G. (2011). 'Becoming somebody': Youth transitions through education and migration in Peru. *Journal of Youth Studies, 14*(4), 395-411.

Dong, X., Chang, E.-S., Wong, E., & Simon, M. (2012). The perceptions, social determinants, and negative health outcomes associated with depressive symptoms among U.S. Chinese older adults. *Gerontologist, 52*(5), 650-663.

Fingerman, K.L., Miller, L.M., Birditt, K.S., & Zarit, S.H. (2009). Giving to the good and the needy: Parental support of grown children. *Journal of Marriage and Family, 71,* 1220-1233.

Fingerman, K.L., VanderDrift, L.E., Dotterer, A.M., Birditt, K.S., & Zarit, S.H. (2011). Support to aging parents and grown children in Black and White families. *The Gerontologist, 51*(4), 441-452.

Hoshino, K. (2012). Sociocultural support model for healthy aging. In A.E. Scharlach & K. Hoshino (Eds.) *Healthy aging in sociocultural context* (pp.86-97). New York: Routledge.

Iwamasa, G.Y., & Iwasaki, M. (2011). A new multidimensional model of successful aging: Perceptions of Japanese American older adults. *Journal of Cross-Cultural Gerontology, 26,* 261-278.

Kim, K., Zarit, S.H., Eggebeen, D.J., Birditt, K.S., & Fingerman, K.L. (2011). Discrepancies in reports of support exchanges between aging parents and their middle-aged children. *The Journals of Gerontology Series B: Psychological Sciences and Social Sciences, 66B*(5), 527-537.

Leinaweaver, J.B. (2010). Kinship paths to and from the New Europe: A unified analysis of Peruvian adoption and migration. *Journal of Latin American and Caribbean Anthropology, 16*(2), 380-400.

National Wellness Institute (2015). Definition of wellness. Retrieved June 20, 2015 from http://www.nationalwellness.org/?page=Six_Dimensions

Roberts, R.E.L., & Bengtson, V.L. (1990). Is intergenerational solidarity a unidimensional construct?: A second test of a formal model. *The Journals of Gerontology: Psychological Sciences and Social Sciences, 45,* S12-S20.

Roberts, R.E.L., & Bengtson, V.L. (1996). Affective ties to parents in early adulthood and self-esteem across 20 years. *Social Psychology Quarterly, 59,* 96-106.

Substance Abuse and Mental Health Services Administration (2015). SAMHSA Wellness Initiative. Retrieved July 12, 2015 from http://www.samhsa.gov/wellness-initiative

School of Public Health, The University of California at Berkeley (2015). History, Retrieved July 12, 2015 from http://sph.berkeley.edu/school/history

Silverstein, M., Gans, D., Lowenstein, A., Giarruso, R., & Bengtson, V.L. (2010). Older parent-child relationships in six developed nations: Comparisons at the intersection of affection and conflict. *Journal of Marriage and Family, 72,* 1006-1021.

Smarbrick, M. (2006). A Wellness Approach, *Psychiatric Rehabilitation Journal, 29*(4), 311-314.

Student Health and Counseling Services, The University of California at Davis (2015). What is wellness? Retrieved June 28, 2015 from https://shcs.ucdavis.edu/

wellness

Tseng W., & Neuhauser, L. (2015). Health Research for Action and Berkeley Wellness Model. Paper presented at the 2015 UC Berkeley International Symposium at Osaka University (Osaka, Japan).

University Health Services, The University of California at Berkeley (2015). Equity, Inclusion, and diversity. Retrieved July 12, 2015 from http://www.uhs.berkeley. edu/home/about/equity.html

University of California at Riverside (2015). UC Living Well. Retrieved from July 12, 2015 from https://welness.ucr.edu/meet_the_team.html

U.S. Census (2014). *2014 National population projections.* New York: U.S. Census Bureau Population Division.

World Health Organization (2015). Definition of health. Retrieved June 28, 2015 from http://www.who.int

Part 1

International Migration and Wellness Innovation in the United States and Sweden

Chapter 1 Cultural Identity and Intergenerational Relationships among Chinese, Japanese, and Peruvian Americans

Kazumi Hoshino, Winston Tseng, Nancy Hikoyeda, & Dolores Gallagher-Thompson

INTRODUCTION

Demographic Changes in the United States

This chapter will examine emotional and social dimensions of wellness and identify how international migration has interacted with wellness among Asian Americans and Hispanic Americans in the United States. Emotional dimension is defined as coping effectively with life and creating satisfying relationships, and social dimension refers to developing a sense of connection, belonging, and a well-developed support system. In this chapter, the authors will analyze intergenerational relationships in terms of emotional dimension, while we will investigate cultural identity with regard to social dimension.

Remarkable demographic changes have occurred in the United States, and the number of Asian Americans has transcended that of Hispanic Americans in 2010 (U.S. Census, 2014). Of those, the six major groups of Asian Americans included Chinese, Indian, Filipino, Korean, Vietnamese, and Japanese Americans (Pew Research Center, 2013). In particular, Chinese Americans, and Japanese Americans showed distinctive trends of immigration patterns and attitudes toward interracial marriage based on each cultural belief such as familism norms and filial piety (Dong, Chang,

Wong, & Simon, 2012; Shibusawa, & Mui, 2001; Iwamasa, & Iwasaki, 2011).

On the other hand, Hispanic Americans have mainly come from Mexico, Peru as well as Central and South America (Pew Research Center, 2013), and Mexicans have mainly immigrated to the United States among Hispanic Americans. Previous studies on health disparities in medical science and social sciences have dominantly focused on Mexican Americans. However, diversity in Hispanic migration has increased, in particular Peruvian Americans. Past research suggested strong intergenerational ties among Peruvian immigrants, based on their cultural and economic backgrounds (Crivello, 2011; Leinaweaver, 2010). Japanese people immigrated to South American countries such as Peru about 100 years ago, and Chinese people have developed China towns in these countries. Therefore, Peruvians have communicated with cultural beliefs and familism norm from China and Japan in their home country as well as in the United States.

It is essential to clarify how Chinese Americans, Japanese Americans, and Peruvian Americans have shaped cultural identity based on their perspectives which have maintained strong intergenerational ties and respect for ancestors. To the best of our knowledge, this is the first study to explore associations between cultural identity and intergenerational relationships and to clarify commonalities and differences of cultural identity and intergenerational relationships among Chinese, Japanese, and Peruvian Americans.

Definition of Cultural Identity

Ethnic identity is defined as an aspect of a person's social identity, "that part of an individual's self-concept which derives from [his/her] knowledge of [his/her] membership in a social group (or groups) together with the value and emotional significance attached to that membership" (Tajfel, 1981, p.255). Erikson (1968, 1980) regarded ethnic identity as a part of identity formation in ethnicity. "The growing child must derive a vitalizing sense of reality from the awareness that his individual ways of mastering experience (his ego synthesis) is a successful variant of a group identity, and is in accord with its space-time and life span" (Erikson, 1980, p.21).

On the other hand, the concept of cultural identity has been widely discussed, and psychometric measurement of cultural identity has been variously developed (Hazuda, Stern, & Haffner, 1998; Mezzich, Ruiperez, Yoon, Liu, & Zapata-Vega, 2009; Friedlander, Friedman, Miller, Ellis, Friedlander, & Mikhaylov, 2010). Cultural identity is defined as an individual's subjective conception of self in relationship to a cultural group(s) (Reber, 1985) that includes ethnicity, race, gender, age, sexual orientation, religion, language, exceptionality, and socioeconomic status. The cultural groups to which people belong can influence the basis for categorization and the formulation of in-groups and out-groups, especially within an institutional context in which cultural groups have differential status and power (Cohen & Lotan, 2004).

"I hypothesize that ethnic, national, and global identifications are developmental in nature and that an individual can attain a healthy and reflective national identification only when he or she has acquired a healthy and reflective cultural identification; and that individuals can develop a reflective and positive global identification only after they have a realistic, reflective, and positive national identification" (Banks, 2006, p.34). These identifications represent stages of cultural identity (including ethnic identity) that consist of six stages: Cultural Psychological Captivity; Cultural

Encapsulation; Cultural Identity Clarification; Biculturalism; Multiculturalism and Reflective Nationalism; and Globalism and Global Competency. In Stage 1 (Cultural Psychological Captivity), the individual does not appear to accept societal and individual beliefs about his/her cultural group and devaluates his/her cultural group and identity. In Stage 2 (Cultural Encapsulation), the individual thinks that his/her cultural group has superiority to other cultural groups and may show negative attitudes towards other groups. In Stage 3 (Cultural Identity Clarification), the individual can clarify his/her identity and accept the positive and negative aspects of his/her cultural group. In Stage 4 (Biculturalism), the individual can participate in his/her own cultural community as well as another cultural community. In Stage 5 (Multiculturalism and Reflective Nationalism), the individual can develop national identity and can work well within several cultures within the nation. In Stage 6 (Globalism and Global Competency), the individual has developed global identities and has enhanced the sensitivity to balance cultural, national, and global identities, and commitments within cultures in his/her nation as well as in other parts of the world (Banks, 2006, pp.138-141). This theory has expanded the influence on the academic areas of education, psychology, public health, broad social and medical sciences, and the educational and clinical practices. The theory also demonstrates a comprehensive and universal perspective that integrates not only individual identification but also national and global identification.

International Migration and Intergenerational Relationships

Previous studies have tried to identify factors that were associated with immigration and assimilation in the United States. Portes, Fernandez-Kelly,

& Haller (2009) presented a model predicting downward assimilation in early adulthood which was composed of human capital, family composition, and modes of incorporation across immigrant generations. School contexts, in particular the students' average statuses have affected the adults' outcomes, and academic achievement as well as educational ambition have limited downward assimilation, reinforcing parental socioeconomic status and intact families. Portes and his colleagues (2009) also demonstrated a model of the process of segmented assimilation which differentiated selective, consonant, and dissonant acculturation among first and second generation immigrants in the contexts of parental human capital, modes of incorporation, and family structure. Authoritative parenting prevented dissonant acculturation, and the presence of significant others, external assistance programs, the preservation of cultural skills, and family memories from home countries led to selective acculturation. These downward assimilation may replicate across generations and strengthen disparities among specific ethnic groups. Fuligni & Masten (2010) reported that expected time spent in work, school, and other relationships had conflict with time spent helping family members. Thus, cultural identity may affect intergenerational relationships among immigrant families.

Theories of intergenerational relationships embraced as the intergenerational stake hypothesis and the intergenerational transmission hypothesis. According to Birditt, Tighe, Fingerman, & Zarit (2012), the intergenerational stake hypothesis, which emerged from Intergenerational Solidarity Theory (Bengtson, & Roberts, 1991; Bengtson, & Schrader, 1982; Silverstein, Gans, Rowenstein, Giarruso, & Bengtson, 2010), suggested that positive feelings such as affection and negative feelings such as conflict varied within families by generation with older generations reporting greater positive quality and lower negative quality than younger generations (Bengtson & Kuypers, 1971). In contrast, family systems theorists proposed that transmission of interaction patterns across generations led to similarities in emotional experience among family members (Bowen, 1978; Fingerman & Bermann, 2000). In terms of intergenerational relationships across three generations, intergenerational relationships among children, adults, and elderly parents were consistent with the intergenerational stake hypothesis and only partially consistent with the intergenerational transmission hypothesis (Birditt, Tighe, Fingerman, & Zarit, 2012). Family generational statuses are associated with intergenerational relationships, and cultural beliefs have a stronger influence on older adults than children and adults among three generations

Bengtson and his colleagues developed Intergenerational Solidarity Theory (Bengtson, & Roberts, 1991; Bengtson, & Schrader, 1982; Silverstein, Gans, Rowenstein, Giarruso, & Bengtson, 2010). The theory classifies intergenerational relationships by combinations of affection/ closeness and conflict (Clarke, Preston, Raskin, & Bengtson, 1999; Silverstein, Gans, Rowenstein, Giarruso, & Bengtson, 2010). Intergenerational relationships among families in diverse countries are categorized as four types of intergenerational relationships: Amicable Type (high closeness and low conflict); Disharmonious Type (low closeness and high conflict); Ambivalent Type (high closeness and high conflict); and Detached Type (low closeness and low conflict). Past studies have confirmed that these types of intergenerational relationships were applicable to diverse ethnic groups based on their international comparative studies on family diversity.

Present Study

The present study will examine cultural identity of children, adults, and elderly parents from the perspectives of first generation Chinese American adults, Japanese American adults, and Peruvian American adults. The study will also analyze the adults' perceived intergenerational relationships between children, adults, and elderly parents. Furthermore, the study will clarify commonalities and differences of cultural identity and intergenerational relationships across the three generations from the perspectives of Chinese adult immigrants, Japanese adult immigrants, and Peruvian adult immigrants.

METHODS

Participants

The sample included 60 participants of Chinese American adults, Japanese American adults, and Peruvian American adults who had at least one child who was born in the United States. They had lived in the United States less than 30 years, and their age ranged from 40 to 59 years old. In-person interviews were conducted in Northern California.

The research project members recruited participants in cooperation with community or church-based organizations in Northern California. The participant was recruited through referrals from presidents of local ethnic community organizations, and distribution of flyers by the research staff or by local ethnic community organizations to their members via online listservs. The flyer was also posted in senior service centers and was handed to the participants at community events.

Interview Survey

In-person interviews were conducted by bilingual/multilingual research project members in English, Spanish, Mandarin, Cantonese, or Japanese using an interview protocol. We adjusted the languages used in each interview was based on the participant's preference, and interviews were held in an interview room at the university or community and church-based organizations, or in their homes in Northern California, based on participants' requests. During the interview, each participant first signed the consent form that indicated agreement of their participation in this research project. Next, participants answered questions concerning demographic variables. Then the interviewers asked adults about cultural identity and intergenerational relationships between children, adults, and elderly parents from perspectives of adults. After the one-hour interview, the participants received compensation ($25) in cash. Mean time of the interviews was 60 minutes. The interviewers also wrote summary field notes of the interviews, including descriptions of the participants such as particular key themes and specific attitudes towards the interviews.

Interview Protocol

Based on Cultural Identity Theory (Banks, 1976, 2006) and Intergenerational Solidarity Theory (Bengtson, & Schrader, 1982; Bengtson, & Roberts, 1991; Roberts, & Bengtson, 1990, 1996; Silverstein, Gans, Lowenstein, Giarusso, & Bengtson, 2010), a new interview protocol was developed in order to estimate cultural identity and intergenerational support exchanges. The Committee for Protection of Human Subjects at the University of California at Berkeley approved this study on research ethnics and legal issues.

RESULTS

Participants' Social Characteristics

The percentage of female participants was 60% among Peruvian American adults, 80% among Chinese American adults, and 90% among Japanese American adults. The mean of years of education was 14.15 years (SD=2.25) among Peruvian American adults, 15.75 years (SD=3.43) among Chinese American adults, and 15.83 years (SD=1.70) among Japanese American adults. The participants who had full-time jobs or part-time jobs were 85% among Peruvian American adults, and each 70% among Chinese American adults and Japanese American adults. The percentage of those who were bilingual in their social lives was 65% among Peruvian American adults, and each 95% among Chinese American adults and Japanese American adults. The mean age of children who were selected by the participants in the interviews was 10.45 years old (SD=6.40) among Peruvian American adults, 18.35 years old (SD=6.39) among Chinese American adults, and 14.55 years old (SD=6.26) among Japanese American adults. The mean age of selected elderly parents was 70.21 years old (SD=8.06) among Peruvian American adults, 75.47 years old (SD=15.96) among Chinese American adults, and 75.90 years old (SD=4.73) among Japanese American adults.

Cultural Identity

A content analysis of the cultural view of the migrant-sending countries revealed six categories among children (Table 1-1), and seven categories among adults (Table 1-2) and elderly parents (Table 1-3): Cultural identity; Linguistic balance; Interpersonal relationships; Social values; Life goals; Religiosity; and Environmental changes. Life goals and the subcategory,

Accomplishments in education and job were found among only adults and elderly parents. With regard to subcategories, Suppressive relationships in Interpersonal relationships was seen among Chinese elderly parents and Japanese elderly parents. Japanese elderly parents also indicated Consideration of others' feelings without words and Keeping homogeneity in Interpersonal relationships as their basic trend.

Eight categories were selected as the cultural view of the migrant-receiving country among children (Table 1-4), adults (Table 1-5), and elderly parents (Table 1-6): Cultural identity; Linguistic balance; Interpersonal relationships; Social values; Life goals; Diversity; and Environmental changes. As for the subcategories, Diversity contained Diverse immigrants (children, adults, and elderly parents), Social integration (adults, and elderly parents), and Multicultural society (adults). Peruvian American children showed Low parental support for children's accomplishments because of financial issues in their family lives, although Peruvian American adults emphasized Helping others. Chinese American adults referred to Too much freedom in Social values and Tiger parents in Life goals. Japanese elderly parents showed No identification of the United States and Living in the home country in Cultural identity.

Chapter 1　Cultural Identity and Intergenerational Relationships among Chinese, Japanese, and Peruvian Americans　27

Table 1-1 The Cultural View of the Migrant-Sending Countries among Children

Categories	Subcategories
1) Cultural Identity	(1) Identity of country origin
	(2) Familiarity with country origin
	(3) Mixed identity
	(4) Analytical view
	(5) No identification of country origin
	(6) Knowledge of only home country
	(7) Generational succession
2) Linguistic balance	(1) Original language use
	(2) Second and third language learning
	(3) Language barriers
3) Interpersonal relationships	(1) Dependent relationships
	(2) Being independent
	(3) Individualism
	(4) Consideration of others' feelings without words
	(5) Respect for parents and older adults
	(6) Suppressive relationships
4) Social values	(1) Materialistic views.
5) Religiosity	(1) Moral
	(2) Religious beliefs.
6) Environmental changes	(1) Socioeconomic environment

Table 1-2 The Cultural View of the Migrant-Sending Countries among Adults

Categories	Subcategories
1) Cultural Identity	(1) Identity of country origin (Familiarity with country origin)
	(2) Mixed identity
	(3) Analytical view
	(4) No identification of country origin
	(5) Knowledge of only home country
	(6) Generational succession
2) Linguistic balance	(1) Original language use
	(2) Second and third language learning
3) Interpersonal relationships	(1) Dependent relationships
	(2) Being independent
	(3) Individualism
	(4) Consideration of others' feelings without words
	(5) Respect for parents and older adults
	(6) Suppressive relationships
	(7) Keeping homogeneity
4) Social values	(1) Materialistic views
5) Life goals	(1) Accomplishments in education and job
6) Religiosity	(1) Moral
	(2) Religious beliefs.
7) Environmental changes	(1)Socioeconomic environment
	(2) Social Security
	(3) Political system
	(4) Educational system.

Table 1-3 The Cultural View of the Migrant-Sending Countries among Elderly Parents

Categories	Subcategories
1) Cultural Identity	(1) Identity of country origin (Familiarity with country origin)
	(2) Mixed identity
	(3) Analytical view
	(4) No identification of country origin
	(5) Knowledge of only home country
	(6) Generational succession
2) Linguistic balance	(1) Original language use
	(2) Second and third language learning
	(3) Language barriers
3) Interpersonal relationships	(1) Dependent relationships
	(2) Being independent
	(3) Individualism
	(4) Consideration of others' feelings without words
	(5) Respect for parents and older adults
	(6) Suppressive relationships
	(7) Keeping homogeneity
4) Social values	(1) Materialistic views
5) Life goals	(1) Accomplishments in education and job
6) Religiosity	(1) Moral
	(2) Religious beliefs
7) Environmental changes	(1) Socioeconomic environment
	(2) Social Security
	(3) Political system
	(4) History (World War Two)
	(5) Natural environment

30   Part 1   International Migration and Wellness Innovation in the United States and Sweden

Table 1-4 The Cultural View of the Migrant-Receiving Country among Children

Categories	Subcategories
1) Cultural Identity	(1) Identity of country origin (Familiarity with country origin)
	(2) Mixed identity
	(3) Analytical view
	(4) No identification of the United States
	(5) Knowledge of only home country
	(6) Living in the home country
	(7) Generational succession
2) Linguistic balance	(1) Original language use
	(2) Second and third language learning
3) Interpersonal relationships	(1) Being independent
	(2) Individualism
	(3) Respect for individuals
	(4) Low Respect for parents, grandparents, and older adults
	(5) Nuclear family centered
4) Religiosity	(1) Moral
	(2) Religious beliefs
5) Social values	(1) Existence of freedom
	(2) Too much freedom
	(3) Organized system
	(4) Helping others
	(5) Discrimination
	(6) Materialistic views
6) Life goals	(1) Accomplishments in education and job
	(2) Accomplishments in marriage
	(3) Tiger parents
	(4) Low parental support for children's accomplishments
	(5) Rational lifestyles
7) Diversity	(1) Diverse immigrants
8) Environmental changes	(1) Socioeconomic environment
	(2) Political system
	(3) Educational system

Chapter 1 Cultural Identity and Intergenerational Relationships among Chinese, Japanese, and Peruvian Americans 31

Table 1-5 The Cultural View of the Migrant-Receiving Country among Adults

Categories	Subcategories
1) Cultural Identity	(1) Identity of country origin (Familiarity with country origin)
	(2) Mixed identity
	(3) Analytical view
	(4) No identification of the United States
	(5) Knowledge of only home country
	(6) Living in the home country
	(7) Generational succession
2) Linguistic balance	(1) Original language use
	(2) Second and third language learning
3) Interpersonal relationships	(1) Being independent
	(2) Individualism
	(3) Respect for individuals
	(4) Low Respect for parents, grandparents, and older adults
	(5) Nuclear family centered
	(6) Friendly relationships
	(7) Superficial relationships
4) Religiosity	(1) Moral
	(2) Religious beliefs
5) Social values	(1) Existence of freedom
	(2) Too much freedom
	(3) Organized system
	(4) Helping others
	(5) Discrimination
	(6) Materialistic views
	(7) Volunteer activities
6) Life goals	(1) Accomplishments in education and job
	(2) Accomplishments in marriage
	(3) Tiger parents
	(4) Low parental support for children's accomplishments
	(5) Rational lifestyles
7) Diversity	(1) Diverse immigrants
	(2) Social integration
	(3) Multicultural society
8) Environmental changes	(1) Socioeconomic environment
	(2) Social Security
	(3) Political system
	(4) International relations
	(5) Educational system
	(6) Health care system

Table 1-6 The Cultural View of the Migrant-Receiving Country among Elderly Parents

Categories	Subcategories
1) Cultural Identity	(1) Identity of country origin (Familiarity with country origin)
	(2) Mixed identity
	(3) Analytical view
	(4) No identification of the United States
	(5) Knowledge of only home country
	(6) Living in the home country
	(7) Generational succession
2) Linguistic balance	(1) Original language use
	(2) Second and third language learning
3) Interpersonal relationships	(1) Being independent
	(2) Individualism
	(3) Respect for individuals
	(4) Low Respect for parents, grandparents, and older adults
	(5) Nuclear family centered
	(6) Friendly relationships
	(7) Superficial relationships
4) Religiosity	(1) Moral
	(2) Religious beliefs
5) Social values	(1) Existence of freedom
	(2) Too much freedom
	(3) Organized system
	(4) Helping others
	(5) Discrimination
	(6) Materialistic views (Emphasis on driving)
	(7) Volunteer activities
6) Life goals	(1) Accomplishments in education and job
	(2) Accomplishments in marriage
	(3) Tiger parents
	(4) Low parental support for children's accomplishments
	(5) Rational lifestyles
7) Diversity	(1) Diverse immigrants
	(2) Social integration
8) Environmental changes	(1) Socioeconomic environment
	(2) Political system
	(3) History (World War Two)
	(4) International relations
	(5) Educational system

Intergenerational Relationships

A content analysis of relationships between children and adults revealed six categories of closeness (Table 1-7) and eight categories of conflict (Table 1-8). Closeness contained the categories: Positive ties; Better relationships; Challenges of appropriate distance in relationships; Average relationships; and Independence of relationships. In terms of subcategories, Japanese American adults emphasized Normal relationships in Average relationships. On the other hand, conflict encompassed the categories: Education; Immigration; Low respect for children; Worse relationships; Cultural differences; Human development; Socioeconomic environment; and Denial of conflict. All groups enlightened Children's higher educational goals in Education. Peruvian American adults focused on Socioeconomic environment, including the subcategories of Social security and Economic development because their home country has had challenges in the unstable political, economic, and societal contexts.

On the other hand, four categories of closeness (Table 1-9) and eight categories of conflict (Table 1-10) were found from a content analysis of relationships between adults and elderly parents. Closeness consisted of the categories: Positive ties; Better relationships; Challenges of appropriate distance in relationships; and Protection against society. Of the subcategories, Peruvian American adults referred to Protection against socioeconomic environment, in which they defended their elderly parents in the United States. Turning to conflict, the categories spanned: Education; Immigration; Low respect for children; Worse relationships; Cultural differences; Human development; Socioeconomic environment; and Denial of conflict. All groups described the subcategory such as Elderly parents' aging, which related to caregiving, and Prolonged conflicts that have occurred from their earlier developmental stages. Peruvian American adults emphasized Socioeconomic environment, including Social security and Economic development, which are central in their conflict.

Table 1-7 Closeness Between Children and Adults

Categories	Subcategories
1) Positive ties	(1) Positive relationships
	(2) Trust
	(3) Advisory role
2) Better relationships	(1) Improving relationships
3) Challenges of appropriate distance in relationships	(1) Low closeness
	(2) Too closeness
5) Average relationships	(1) Normal relationships
6) Independence of relationships	(1) Independent relationships

Table 1-8 Conflict Between Children and Adults

Categories	Subcategories
1) Education	(1) Higher educational goals
2) Immigration	(1) Immigration and geographic mobility
3) Low respect for children	(1) Low respect for children
	(2) Too much support to children
4) Worse relationships	(1) Degenerating relationships
	(2) Low communication
5) Cultural differences	(1) Cultural backgrounds
	(2) Linguistic barriers
6) Human development	(1) Adults' aging
	(2) Differences of developmental stages
7) Socioeconomic environment	(1) Economic development
	(2) Social security
8) Denial of conflicts	(1) Denial of conflicts

Chapter 1 Cultural Identity and Intergenerational Relationships among Chinese, Japanese, and Peruvian Americans   35

Table 1-9 Closeness Between Adults and Elderly Parents

Categories	Subcategories
1) Positive ties	(1) Positive relationships
	(2) Trust
	(3) Advisory role
2) Better relationships	(1) Improving relationships
3) Challenges of appropriate distance in relationships	(1) Low closeness
	(2) Too closeness
4) Protection against society	(1) Protection against socioeconomic development
	(1) Independent relationships

Table 1-10 Conflict Between Adults and Elderly Parents

Final Categories	Previous Categories
1) Education	(1) Higher educational goals
2) Immigration	(1) Immigration and geographic mobility
3) Low respect for adults	(1) Low respect for adults
	(2) Too much support to adults
4) Worse relationships	(1) Degenerating relationships
	(2) Low communication
5) Cultural differences	(1) Cultural backgrounds
	(2) Ambivalence
6) Human development	(1) Elderly parents' aging
	(2) Differences of developmental stages
	(3) Prolonged conflicts
7) Socioeconomic environment	(1) Economic development
	(2) Social security
8) Denial of conflicts	(1) Denial of conflicts

DISCUSSION

Our findings showed that Immigration, adults' expectations of children's higher educational achievement in Education, Adults' aging, Differences of developmental stages, and Socioeconomic environment related to conflict between children and adults. Also, Immigration, Elderly parents' aging, Prolonged conflict, Elderly parents' low respect for adults, and Socioeconomic environment affected relationships between adults and elderly parents. In particular, Peruvian American adults emphasized Socioeconomic environment and strengthened generational reciprocity in terms of higher expectations of children's educational achievement and professional jobs by reflecting their familism norms and unstable socioeconomic status in the United States and Peru. To support children's education, adults and elderly parents work hard and sometimes may lose respectful communication with children. Thus, our findings support previous studies (Crivello, 2011; Leinaweaver, 2010) and further demonstrate strong intergenerational reciprocity among Peruvian American adults, Peruvian American children, and Peruvian elderly parents.

Chinese American adults also had stronger motivations for children's successful career like Tiger parents and showed concerns of social values such as Too much freedom in the United States. Japanese American adults endorsed existence of freedom and questioned interpersonal relationships such as Consideration of others' feelings without words in Japan. However, since elderly parents living in Japan might not understand such sociocultural differences, Japanese American adults perceived Elderly parents' low respect for adults and Ambivalence. In addition, depending on the level of acculturation, some of Chinese American adults and Japanese American adults are accommodated to a mainstream American culture, while others have still maintained their home countries' cultural practices and beliefs. These findings coincide to other work (Iwasaki & Iwamasa, 2011; Shibusawa & Mui, 2001; Dong et al., 2012; Tsai, Ying, & Lee, 2000; Ying, Lee, &Tsai, 2007). Thus, Peruvian American adults are more likely to strengthen their cultural heritage across three generations, although some of Chinese American adults and Japanese American adults, and their children tend to adopt the local culture in the United States according to their acculturation.

This study has a few limitations. First, each sample was small in California, and so researchers need to use a population-based sample in other states to confirm our findings. Second, as this study conducted interviews with only adults, further interviews are expected to ask their children and elderly parents for their perspectives. Third, questions assessing cultural identity in the interview protocol may be added to evaluate participants' cultural beliefs for several cultures more accurately, while the current two items assessing cultural identity can evaluate cultural beliefs for both cultures of immigrant-sending and receiving countries.

ACKNOWLEDGMENTS

This study was partly presented at the 75th Annual Scientific Meeting of the Gerontological Society of America in San Diego (Hoshino, Tseng, Hikoyeda, Gallagher-Thompson, Ventura, & Inoue, 2012). The authors appreciate Dr. S. Leonard Syme and Dr. Winston Tseng who allow us to conduct this research at the University of California at Berkeley. The authors also wish to thank Dr. Andrew E. Scharlach for his valuable suggestions as a research consultant. Moreover, the authors acknowledge the participants, community-based organizations, and the research assistants, in particular Mr. Jomer Ventura and Ms. Hazuki Inoue. This study was supported by the Foundation of the Japanese Certification Board for Clinical Psychologists to Kazumi Hoshino.

REFERENCES

Banks, J. (1976). The emerging stages of ethnicity: Implications for staff development. *Educational Leadership, 34*(3), 190-193.

Banks, J. (2006). *Cultural diversity and education: Foundations, curriculum, and teaching (5 th ed.).* Boston: Pearson Education.

Bengtson, V.L., & Kuypers, J. (1971). Generational difference and the developmental stake. *International Journal of Aging and Human Development, 2,* 249-260.

Bengtson, V.L., & Roberts, R.E.L. (1991). Intergenerational solidarity in aging families: An example of formal theory construction. *Journal of Marriage and Family, 53,* 856-870.

Bengtson, V.L., & Schrader, S.S. (1982). Parent-child relations. In D. Mangen & W. Peterson (Eds.) *Handbook of research instruments in social gerontology* (pp.115-185). Minneapolis: University of Minnesota Press.

Birditt, K.S., Tighe, L.A., Zarit, S.H., & Fingerman, K.L. (2012). Intergenerational relationships quality across three generations. *The Journals of Gerontology Series B: Psychological Sciences and Social Sciences, 67B*(5), 627-638.

Bowen, M. (1978). *Family therapy in clinical practice.* Northvale, NJ: Jason Aronson Inc.

Clarke, E.J., Preston, M., Raskin, J., & Bengtson, V.L. (1999). Types of conflicts and tensions between older parents and adult children. *Gerontologist, 39,* 261-270.

Cohen, E.G., & Lotan, R.A. (2004). Equity in heterogeneous classrooms. In J.A. Banks & C.A.M. Banks (Eds.) *Handbook of research on multicultural education* (pp.736-750). San Francisco: Jossey-Bass.

Crivello, G. (2011). 'Becoming somebody': Youth transitions through education and migration in Peru. *Journal of Youth Studies, 14*(4), 395-411.

Dong, X., Chang, E.-S., Wong, E., & Simon, M. (2012). The perceptions, social determinants, and negative health outcomes associated with depressive symptoms among U.S. Chinese older adults. *Gerontologist, 52*(5), 650-663.

Erikson, E.H. (1968). *Identity: Youth and crisis.* New York: W. W. Norton & Company.

Erikson, E.H. (1980). *Identity and the life cycle.* New York: W. W. Norton & Company.

Fingerman, K.L., & Bermann, E. (2000). Applications of family systems theory to the study of adulthood. *International Journal of Aging and Human Development, 51*, 5-29.

Fingerman, K.L., Miller, L.M., Birditt, K.S., & Zarit, S.H. (2009). Giving to the good and the needy: Parental support of grown children. *Journal of Marriage and Family, 71*, 1220-1233.

Fingerman, K.L., VanderDrift, L.E., Dotterer, A.M., Birditt, K.S., & Zarit, S.H. (2011). Support to aging parents and grown children in Black and White families. *The Gerontologist, 51*(4), 441-452.

Friedlander, M.L., Friedman, M.L., Miller, M.J., Ellis, M.V., Friedlander, L.K., & Mikhaylov, V.G. (2010). Introducing a brief measure of cultural and religious identification in American Jewish identity. *Journal of Counseling Psychology, 57*(3), 345-360.

Fuligni, A., & Masten, C.L. (2010). Daily family interactions among young adults in the United States from Latin American, Filipino, East Asian, and European backgrounds. *International Journal of Ethnic and Migration Studies, 34*(6), 491-499.

Hazuda, H.P., Stern, M.P., & Haffner, S. M. (1998). Acculturation and assimilation among Mexican Americans: Scales and population-based data. *Social Science Quarterly, 68*, 687-706, Austin: University of Texas Press

Hoshino, K., Tseng, W., Hikoyeda, N., Gallagher-Thompson, D., Ventura, J., & Inoue, H. (2012). Cultural identity and intergenerational relationships among Latino and Asian Americans. Poster presented at the 75th Annual Scientific Meeting of the Gerontological Society of America (San Diego, USA).

Iwamasa, G.Y., & Iwasaki, M. (2011). A new multidimensional model of successful aging: Perceptions of Japanese American older adults. *Journal of Cross-Cultural Gerontology, 26*, 261-278.

Mezzich, J.E., Ruiperez, M.A., Yoon, G., Liu, J., & Zapata-Vega, M.I. (2009). Measuring cultural identity: Validation of a modified Cortes, Rogler and Malgady Bicultural Scale in three ethnic groups in New York. *Culture, Medicine, and Psychiatry, 33*, 451-472.

Pew Research Center (2013). *The rise of Asian Americans.* Washington, DC: Pew Research Center.

Portes, A., Fernandez-Kelly, P., & Haller, W. (2009). The adaptation of the immigrant second generation in America: A theoretical overview and recent evidence. *Journal of Ethnic and Migration Studies, 35*(7), 1077-1104.

Silverstein, M., Gans, D., Lowenstein, A., Giarruso, R., & Bengtson, V.L. (2010). Older parent-child relationships in six developed nations: Comparisons at the intersection of affection and conflict. *Journal of Marriage and Family, 72*, 1006-1021.

Tsai, J.L., Ying, Y.-W., & Lee, P.A. (2000). The meaning of "being Chinese" and "being American" variation among Chinese American young adults. *Journal of Cross-Cultural Psychology, 31*(3), 302-332.

U.S. Census (2014). *2014 National population projections*. New York: U.S. Census Bureau Population Division.

Ying, Y.-W., Lee, P.A., & Tsai, J.L. (2007). Predictors of depressive symptoms in Chinese American college students: Parent and peer attachment, college challenges, and sense of coherence. *American Journal of Orthopsychiatry, 77*(2), 316-323.

Chapter 2　Cultural Identity and Intergenerational Support among Asian and Hispanic Americans

Kazumi Hoshino, Winston Tseng, Nancy Hikoyeda, & Dolores Gallagher-Thompson

INTRODUCTION

Cultural Identity and Intergenerational Support

Chapter 2 will analyze cultural identity and intergenerational support as social dimension of wellness among Chinese Americans, Japanese Americans, and Peruvian Americans in the United States. The authors will also examine associations between cultural identity, intergenerational support, and intergenerational relationship among the three groups. Finally, the authors will demonstrate a new model of cultural identity, intergenerational support, and intergenerational relationship, which is derived from emotional dimension of wellness, based on a content analysis of the interview data.

　　Transitions in family diversity have influenced intergenerational support worldwide. Intergenerational support is affected by beliefs of family obligations, cultural identity, ethnicity, immigrant generations, and years of residence in the United States (Phinney, 1992; Phinney, & Tanya, 2000; Juang, & Nguyen, 2010). Beliefs of family obligation had a stronger influence on African American adults than European American adults in family support exchanges between grown children and adults as well as between adults and aging parents (Fingerman, VanderDrift, Dotterer, Birditt, &

Zarit, 2011). Adult children among European and African Americans reported that they provided support more than their parents reported receiving, and that they showed differences in the types of support from parents to adult children (Kim, Zarit, Eggebeen, Birditt, & Fingerman, 2011). Such discrepancies were associated with parents' family obligation expectations and each individual cultural identity.

Fingerman et al. (2011) pointed out that European Americans provided more support to grown children than African Americans, and African Americans provided more support to elderly parents than European Americans. The former was associated with grown children's postponed transition from adolescence to young adulthood, and the latter occurred due to longer life expectancy. In addition, even in East Asian countries, which have been considered ethnically homogenous, voluntary-based support exchanges between adult daughters and elderly mothers have gradually become more salient than obligatory-based support exchanges between daughters-in-law and elderly parents-in law, in particular in urban areas (Kim, Zarit, & Han, 2011: Arai, Zarit, Sugiura, & Washio, 2002; Arai, 2000; Arai & Ikegami, 1998).

However, Hispanic Americans and Latino Americans have maintained obligatory intergenerational support exchanges as a mutual responsibility of family members to survive in migrant receiving countries and to establish financial security. Peruvian immigrants, in particular adults and elderly parents, who have experienced a lack of sufficient resources in Peru, have higher expectations that children should obtain higher education and better jobs in order to escape from poverty (Crivello, 2011). Also, Peruvians hold stronger beliefs that they should expand their support not only for parents and grandparents but also for siblings and relatives, once immigrants

Chapter 2 Cultural Identity and Intergenerational Support among Asian and Hispanic Americans   43

establish more stable financial lives in migrant receiving countries than their lives in the country of origin (Leinaweaver, 2010).

Cultural Identity, Intergenerational Relationships, and Intergenerational Support

On the other hand, cultural identity and intergenerational support each relate to intergenerational relationships as well. Intergenerational Solidarity Theory classifies intergenerational relationships by affection/closeness and conflict, based on historical, societal, and policy relevant backgrounds (Bengtson, & Schrader, 1982; Bengtson, & Roberts, 1991; Silverstein, Gans, Lowenstein, Giarusso, & Bengtson, 2010). Relationships between young adults and their parents also affected intergenerational support and influenced cultural identity among Chinese Americans (Juang, & Nguyen, 2010). In addition, middle aged couples were less likely to have traditional patterns of support between adults and aging parents, which emphasized the relationship with husband's parents in South Korea (Kim, Zarit, & Han, 2011), while couples with non-traditional exchange patterns with parents had better marital relationships than did couples whose exchanges with parents derived from obligatory norms. King, Ledwell, and Pearce-Morris (2013) also suggested that adult children who participated in religious activities were more likely to give support to their parents and developed more positive relationships than their counterpart. King and his colleagues (2013) concluded religiosity was associated with intergenerational relationships and well-being of both generations.

In reviewing the previous studies, the important question of how cultural identity, intergenerational support, and intergenerational relationships related has not been identified, in particular among Hispanic

44   Part 1   International Migration and Wellness Innovation in the United States and Sweden

Americans and Asian Americans in the United States who have been enlightened from the perspective of the distinguished demographic changes. Therefore, it is a crucial agenda to understand relationships between the three variables, which link to well-being and aging well.

Present Study

Although previous studies reported associations between cultural identity, intergenerational support, and intergenerational relationships, it is not clear how these variables have interacted with each other. Family transitions to non-traditional intergenerational relationships also have variations in Hispanic Americans and Asian Americans, in particular underrepresented populations.

The present study will examine cultural identity and intergenerational support between adults, their children, and their elderly parents among Chinese Americans, Japanese Americans, and Peruvian Americans in the United States that reflect current trends of underrepresented populations of Hispanic Americans and Asian Americans. The authors will also propose a new model of cultural identity, intergenerational support, and intergenerational relationships in terms of a content analysis of the interview data.

METHODS

Participants

Sixty participants included, 20 Chinese, 20 Japanese, and 20 Peruvian first generation adult immigrants (the age range= 40-59 years old). The participants had lived in the United States less than 30 years and had at least one child who was born in the United States. They were recruited in partnership with community-based organizations in the San Francisco Bay Area.

Interview Survey

Bilingual researchers conducted in-person interviews in English, Spanish, Mandarin, Cantonese, or Japanese, depending on the participants' language preferences at the university, community-based organizations, or their homes. The interviewers asked adults about cultural identity and intergenerational support, by using a semi-structured interview protocol based on Cultural Identity Theory (Banks, 2006) and Intergenerational Solidarity Theory (Bengtson, & Roberts, 1991; Bengtson, & Schrader, 1982; Silverstein, Gans, Rowenstein, Giarruso, & Bengtson, 2010).

Data Analysis

This study conducted a content analysis. A research member rated all data, and another research member analyzed one-third of the data. The percentage of inter-rater consistency of a content analysis was 86%.

RESULTS

Participants' Social Characteristics

The mean of the participants' years of education of Peruvian American adults was 14.15 years (SD=2.25), that of Chinese American adults was 15.75 years (SD=3.43), and that of Japanese American adults was 15.83 years (SD=1.70). The percentage of those with full-time or part-time jobs of Peruvian American adults was 85%, while Chinese American adults and

Japanese American adults was 70%. The mean age of Peruvian American children who were selected by the participants in the interviews was 10.45 years old (SD=6.40), that of Chinese American children was 18.35 years old (SD=6.39), and that of Japanese American children was 14.55 years old (SD=6.26). The mean age of selected Peruvian elderly parents was 70.21 years old (SD=8.06), that of Chinese elderly parents was 75.47 years old (SD=15.96), and that of Japanese elderly parents was 75.90 years old (SD=4.73).

Cultural Identity

Six categories were found among children, and seven categories were seen among elderly parents and adults via a content analysis of a cultural view of migrant-sending countries, including Cultural identity, Linguistic balance, Interpersonal relationships, Social values, Life goals, Religiosity, and Environmental changes. Only elderly parents and adults showed an additional subcategory in Life goals, such as Accomplishments in education and job. Chinese elderly parents and Japanese elderly parents referred to Suppressive relationships in Interpersonal relationships. Japanese elderly parents also indicated Consideration of others' feelings without words and Keeping homogeneity.

Children, elderly parents, and adults were analyzed as having eight categories as a cultural view of the migrant receiving country, including Cultural identity, Linguistic balance, Interpersonal relationships, Social values, Life goals, Diversity, and Environmental changes. Diversity had subcategories such as Diverse immigrants, Social integration, and Multicultural society, although only adults referred to the latter two subcategories. Peruvian American adults preferred Helping others however,

Low parental support for children's accomplishments was found among Peruvian American children. Chinese American adults referred to Too much freedom in Social values and Tiger parents in Life goals. Japanese elderly parents showed No identification of the United States and Living in the home country in Cultural identity.

Intergenerational Support between Children and Adults

As Table 2-1 shows, eleven categories and subcategories were selected as adults' expectations of providing support for children: Full support; Educational support; Information support; Emotional support; Financial support; Instrumental support; Caring; Religious support; Being independent; Being professionals; and No expectation. Twelve categories and the subcategories were selected as adults' beliefs of providing support for children (Table 2-2). Of those, ten categories were as same as adults' expectations, and two other categories were Generational reciprocity and No belief.

Adults' expectations of receiving support from children had eleven categories and subcategories: Educational support; Information support; Emotional support; Financial support; Instrumental support; Caring; Religious support; Being independent; Being professionals; Future caregiving for adults; and No expectation (Table 2-3). Adults' beliefs of receiving support from children had twelve categories and subcategories (Table 2-4). Ten categories were the same as those of adults' expectations of receiving support from children, and two other categories were Generational reciprocity and No belief. Remarkably, adults' expectations of receiving support from children included Generational reciprocity, while adults' beliefs of receiving support from children contained not only

Table 2-1 Adults' Expectations: Providing Support for Children

Final Categories	Previous Categories
1) Full support	Full support.
2) Educational support	Educational support; Linguistic support; Educational accomplishments.
3) Information support	Information support.
4) Emotional support	Emotional support; More emotional support; Unconditional love; Mental support; Communication; Trust; Feeling pain: Protection against discrimination
5) Financial support	Financial support.
6) Instrumental support	Instrumental support; Assistance of household chores; Companionship.
7) Caring	Caring.
8) Religious support	Religious support: Moral support; Religious succession.
9) Being independent	Being independent.
10) Being professionals	Being professionals.
11) No expectation	No expectation

Chapter 2 Cultural Identity and Intergenerational Support among Asian and Hispanic Americans   49

Table 2-2 Adults' Beliefs: Providing Support for Children

Final Categories	Previous Categories
1) Full support	Full support.
2) Educational support	Educational support; Linguistic support; Educational accomplishments.
3) Information support	Information support.
4) Emotional support	Emotional support; More emotional support; Unconditional love; Mental support; Communication; Trust; Feeling pain; Respect for children.
5) Financial support	Financial support.
6) Instrumental support	Instrumental support; Assistance of household chores; Companionship.
7) Caring	Caring.
8) Religious support	Religious support: Moral support; Religious succession.
9) Being independent	Being independent.
10) Being professionals	Being professionals.
11) Generational reciprocity	Generational reciprocity.
12) No belief	No belief.

Table 2-3 Adults' Expectations: Receiving Support from Children

Final Categories	Previous Categories
1) Educational support	Educational support; Linguistic support; Educational accomplishments.
2) Information support	Information support.
3) Emotional support	Emotional support; More emotional support; Unconditional love; Mental support; Communication; Trust; Feeling pain; Protection against discrimination.
4) Financial support	Financial support.
5) Instrumental support	Instrumental support; Assistance of household chores; Companionship.
6) Caring	Caring.
7) Religious support	Religious support; Moral support; Religious succession.
8) Being independent	Being independent.
9) Being professionals	Being professionals.
10) Future caregiving for adults	Future Caregiving for adults.
11) No expectation	No expectation; Partners' role.

Chapter 2 Cultural Identity and Intergenerational Support among Asian and Hispanic Americans 51

Table 2-4 Adults' Beliefs: Receiving Support from Children

Final Categories	Previous Categories
1) Educational support	Educational support; Linguistic support; Educational accomplishments.
2) Information support	Information support.
3) Emotional support	Emotional support; More emotional support; Unconditional love; Mental support; Communication; Trust; Feeling pain: Protection against discrimination; Respect for parents.
4) Financial support	Financial support.
5) Instrumental support	Instrumental support; Assistance of household chores; Companionship.
6) Caring	Caring.
7) Religious support	Religious support: Moral support; Religious succession.
8) Being independent	Being independent.
9) Being professionals	Being professionals.
10) Future caregiving for adults	Future Caregiving for adults.
11) Generational reciprocity	Generational reciprocity.
12) No belief	No belief.

52   Part 1   International Migration and Wellness Innovation in the United States and Sweden

Generational reciprocity but also Future caregiving for adults. However, some participants of Chinese Americans and Japanese Americans also emphasized No expectation and No belief.

Intergenerational Support between Adults and Elderly Parents

The following thirteen categories and subcategories were selected as adults' expectations of providing support for elderly parents: Educational support; Information support; Emotional support; Financial support; Instrumental support; Caring; Religious support; Being independent; Being professionals; Caregiving for elderly parents; Familism norms; Voluntary support relationships between mothers and daughters; and No expectation (Table 2-5). Adults' beliefs of providing support for elderly parents consisted of thirteen categories and subcategories (Table 2-6). Eleven categories were as same as those of adults' expectations of providing support for elderly parents, and two other categories were Adults' family priority and No belief. No expectation included the subcategory, Community support, while No belief contained National health care policy for elderly care.

Twelve categories and the subcategories were revealed in adults' expectations of receiving support from elderly parents: Educational support; Information support; Emotional support; Financial support; Instrumental support; Caring; Religious support; Being independent; Caregiving for adults; Familism norms; Support grandchildren; and No expectation (Table 2-7). No expectation contained the subcategory, Community support. On the other hand, adults' beliefs of receiving support from elderly parents had thirteen categories and the subcategories (Table 2-8). Ten categories were as same as those of adults' expectation of receiving support from elderly parents, and three other categories were Generational reciprocity,

Chapter 2 Cultural Identity and Intergenerational Support among Asian and Hispanic Americans 53

Table 2-5 Adults' Expectations: Providing Support for Elderly Parents

Final Categories	Previous Categories
1) Educational support	Educational support; Linguistic support; Educational accomplishments.
2) Information support	Information support.
3) Emotional support	Emotional support; More emotional support; Unconditional love; Mental support; Communication; Trust; Feeling pain.
4) Financial support	Financial support.
5) Instrumental support	Instrumental support; Assistance of household chores; Companionship.
6) Caring	Caring.
7) Religious support	Religious support: Moral support; Religious succession.
8) Being independent	Being independent; Being dependent.
9) Being professionals	Being professionals.
10) Caregiving for elderly parents	Future Caregiving for elderly parents; Direct caregiving; Arrangement of caregiving.
11) Familism norms	Familism norms.
12) Voluntary support relationships between mothers and daughters	Voluntary support relationships between mothers and daughters between mothers and daughters
13) No expectation	No expectation; Community support.

Table 2-6 Adults' Beliefs: Providing Support for Elderly Parents

Final Categories	Previous Categories
1) Educational support	Educational support; Linguistic support; Educational accomplishments.
2) Information support	Information support.
3) Emotional support	Emotional support; More emotional support; Unconditional love; Mental support; Communication; Trust; Feeling pain.
4) Financial support	Financial support.
5) Instrumental support	Instrumental support; Assistance of household chores; Companionship.
6) Caring	Caring.
7) Religious support	Religious support: Moral support; Religious succession.
8) Being independent	Being independent; Being dependent.
9) Being professionals	Being professionals.
10) Caregiving for elderly parents	Future Caregiving for elderly parents; Direct caregiving; Arrangement of caregiving.
11) Familism norms	Familism norms; Filial piety.
12) Adults' family priority	Adults' family priority.
13) No belief	No belief; National health policy for elderly care.

Chapter 2   Cultural Identity and Intergenerational Support among Asian and Hispanic Americans   55

Table 2-7 Adults' Expectations: Receiving Support from Elderly Parents

Category	Subcategory
1) Educational support	Educational support; Linguistic support; Educational accomplishments.
2) Information support	Information support.
3) Emotional support	Emotional support; More emotional support; Unconditional love; Mental support; Communication; Trust; Feeling pain.
4) Financial support	Financial support.
5) Instrumental support	Instrumental support; Assistance of household chores; Companionship.
6) Caring	Caring.
7) Religious support	Religious support: Moral support; Religious succession.
8) Being independent	Being independent.
9) Caregiving for adults	Caregiving for adults.
10) Familism norms	Familism norms
11) Support grandchildren	Support grandchildren.
12) No expectation	No expectation; Community support.

Table 2-8 Adults' Beliefs: Receiving Support from Elderly Parents

Final Categories	Previous Categories
1) Educational support	Educational support; Linguistic support; Educational accomplishments.
2) Information support	Information support.
3) Emotional support	Emotional support; More emotional support; Unconditional love; Mental support; Communication; Trust; Feeling pain; Respect for adults.
4) Financial support	Financial support.
5) Instrumental support	Instrumental support; Assistance of household chores; Companionship.
6) Caring	Caring.
7) Religious support	Religious support: Moral support; Religious succession.
8) Being independent	Being independent; Being dependent.
9) Caregiving for adults	Caregiving for adults.
10) Familism norms	Familism norms.
11) Generational reciprocity	Generational reciprocity; Support grandchildren; Adults' supportive roles.
12) Voluntary support relationships between mothers and daughters	Voluntary support relationships between mothers and daughters.
13) No belief	No belief.

Voluntary relationships between mothers and daughters; and No belief.

A Model of Cultural Identity, Intergenerational Support, and Intergenerational Relationships

As Figure 2-1 shows, the present study demonstrates a new Model of Cultural Identity, Intergenerational Support, and Intergenerational Relationships, based on categories and subcategories in terms of a content analysis. Cultural identity, intergenerational support, and intergenerational relationships are affected by demographic variables such as age, gender, education, current job, socioeconomic status, language proficiency, immigrant generation, and migration patterns.

Chinese American adults, Japanese American adults, and Peruvian American adults of first generation immigrants understand categories and subcategories of cultural identity, including Diversity, Socioeconomic environment, Religiosity, Social values such as Social policy for elderly care, Political system, and History in addition to Interpersonal relationships, and Linguistic balance. They also recognize commonalities and differences of cultural identity across three generations. Such aspects relate to intergenerational support between adults and their children as well as between adults and their elderly parents. Cultural norms such as Generational reciprocity and Familism norms, as well as Family transitions like Voluntary support relationships between mothers and daughters correlate to intergenerational support exchanges. Furthermore, associations of cultural identity and intergenerational support relate to intergenerational relationships between adults, their children, and their elderly parents formed by closeness and conflict.

Demographic variables: Age; Sex; Education; Current Job; Socioeconomic status; Immigrant generation; Language proficiency; Migration patterns.

↓   Intergenerational

Adults'Cultural identity: → Intergenerational support ← Children's Cultural identity: ⇒ relationships

Linguistic balance;	Linguistic balance;	Closeness:
Interpersonal relationships;	Interpersonal relationships;	Positive ties;
Social values;	Social values;	Better relationships;
Life goals; Religiosity;	Life goals; Religiosity;	Challenges of appropriate
Environmental changes;	Environmental changes.	distance in relationships;
Diversity.		Average relationships;

→ Providing support for children →   Independence of
Adults' expectations/beliefs   relationships.
← Receiving support from children ←   Conflict: Education;
Adults' expectations/beliefs   Immigration;
↑   ↑   Low respect for children;

Voluntary support relationships   Cultural norms: Worse relationships;
between mothers and daughters   Generational reciprocity; Familism norms.   Cultural differences;
        Human development;
        Socioeconomic environment.

↓   ↑

                                                                        Intergenerational

Adults'Cultural identity: → Intergenerational support ← Elderly parents'
Cultural ⇒ relationships
identity: Closeness: Positive ties;

Linguistic balance;	Linguistic balance;	Better relationships;
Interpersonal relationships;	Interpersonal relationships;	Challenges of appropriate
Social values;	Social values;	distance in relationships;
Life goals;	Life goals;	Average relationships;
Religiosity;	Religiosity;	Protection against society.
Environmental changes;	Environmental changes.	Conflict: Education;
Diversity.		Immigration;

→ Providing support for elderly parents →   Low respect for adults;
Adults' expectations/beliefs   Worse relationships;
↑   ↑   Cultural differences;

Voluntary support relationships   Cultural norms: Human development;
between mothers and daughters   Generational reciprocity; Familism norms.   Socioeconomic environment.

↓

← Receiving support from elderly parents ←
Adults' expectations/beliefs
↑

Cultural norms:
Generational reciprocity; Familism norms.

Figure 2-1. A Model of Cultural Identity, Intergenerational Support, and Intergenerational Relationships

DISCUSSION

The present study examined cultural identity, intergenerational support, and intergenerational relationships among Chinese American adults, Japanese American adults, and Peruvian American adults, according to a qualitative data analysis. With regard to intergenerational support between children and adults, Peruvian American adults indicated Generational reciprocity that they should provide support for children, and that children should provide support for adults. Some Chinese American adults and Japanese American adults expected, based on Familism norms that they would receive caregiving from children when they need in the future. However, Chinese American adults and Japanese American adults who had grown children showed No expectation and No belief of providing support for children as well as receiving support from children. They understand that they obtained benefits of individualism and freedom in the United States, and that they should respect children's rights, even if they need caregiving in the future.

In terms of intergenerational support between adults and elderly parents, Peruvian American adults indicated Generational reciprocity that they should provide support for elderly parents, and that elderly parents should provide support for adults. This is because Peruvian American adults, Peruvian American children, and Peruvian elderly parents need to establish financial stability in the United States in which such trends are affected by their circular migration patterns, and our findings coincide with previous work (Crivello, 2011; Leinaweaver, 2010). Some Chinese American adults and Japanese American adults kept Familism norms and expected that they should support caregiving for elderly parents in their capability.

However, Chinese American adults and Japanese American adults also indicated No expectation as well as No belief, and they aimed at Voluntary-based relationships between mothers and daughters rather than obligatory relationships. Our findings support family transitions and increasing family diversity (Fingerman et al., 2011; Kim et al., 2011, 2012). They also acknowledged the importance of social policy for elderly care instead of family caregiving.

A new Model of Cultural Identity, Intergenerational Support, and Intergenerational Relationships integrates individual cultural beliefs, support exchanges, and relationships between adults, their children, and their elderly parents formed by closeness and conflict, based on demographic variables. The authors also incorporate these individual variables into societal variables such as societal cultural scheme, social policy, political system, and history in the model. As Silverstein et al. (2010) suggested, societal factors have shaped family relationships and varied dominant family types in comparative studies in the United States and Europe. Thus, the authors demonstrate a unique model of cultural identity, intergenerational support, and intergenerational relationships from a content analysis which spans important variables in the levels of individual, family, and society.

The present study limits a generalizability of these outcomes because of a small sample that included only adults. Future research needs to use national representative data of children, adults, and elderly parents. Also, we should explore other relevant variables such as spirituality. Goins, Spencer, McGuire, Goldberg, Wen, and Henderson (2010) found that identification with native identity, native language use, and cultural identity (i.e., participation in ethnic events) and spirituality (i.e., engagement in traditional healing practices) were positively related to their intergenerational support among American Indians. Lewis (2011) also reported that Alaska Natives represented culturally-specific successful aging, including cultural identity (i.e., engagement in ethnic roles such as traditional leaders), intergenerational support in their communities (i.e., providing wisdom and experiences for younger generations), and spirituality.

However, our findings accurately respond to specific cultural and generational needs among first generation adult immigrants, whereas previous studies mainly focused on Mexican Americans among Hispanic Americans as well as older Chinese Americans, and older Japanese Americans. This study also contributes to clarify associations between cultural identity, intergenerational support, and intergenerational relationships among Chinese, Japanese, and Peruvian Americans of first generation immigrants.

ACKNOWLEDGMENTS

This study was partly presented at the 75th Annual Scientific Meeting of the Gerontological Society of America (Tseng, Hoshino, Hikoyeda, Gallagher-Thompson, Inoue, & Ventura, 2012). The authors acknowledge Dr. S. Leonard Syme and Dr. Winston Tseng to support this research. The authors also wish to thank Dr. Andrew E. Scharlach for his comments as a research consultant. Furthermore, the authors appreciate participants, community-based organizations, and research assistants, including Mr. Jomer Ventura and Ms. Hazuki Inoue. This study was supported by the Foundation of the Japanese Certification Board for Clinical Psychologists

(Principal Investigator: Kazumi Hoshino).

REFERENCES

Arai, Y. (2000). Challenges of an aging society in Japan. *Registered Home and Services, 4*(12), 182-184.

Arai, Y., & Ikegami, N. (1998). How will Japan cope with the impending surge of dementia? In A.W.B. Winblad, B. Jonsson, & G. Karlson (Eds.) *The health economics of dementia.* Chichester: Wiley.

Arai, Y., Zarit, S.H., Sugiura, M., & Washio, M. (2002). Patterns of outcome of caregiving for the impaired elderly: A longitudinal study in Japan. *Aging and Mental Health, 6*, 39-46.

Banks, J. A. (1976). The emerging stages of ethnicity: Implications for staff development. *Educational Leadership, 34* (3), 190-193.

Banks, J. A. (2006). *Cultural diversity and education: Foundations, curriculum, and teaching* (5th ed.). Boston: Pearson Education.

Bengtson, V.L., & Roberts, R.E.L. (1991). Intergenerational solidarity in aging families: An example of formal theory construction. *Journal of Marriage and Family, 53*, 856-870.

Bengtson, V.L., & Schrader, S.S. (1982). Parent-child relations. In D. Mangen & W. Peterson (Eds.) *Handbook of research instruments in social gerontology* (pp.115-185). Minneapolis: University of Minnesota Press.

Cheng, S.-T., Li, K.-K., Leung, E.M.F., & Chan, A.C.M. (2011). Social exchanges and subjective well-being: Do sources of positive and negative exchanges matter? *The Journals of Gerontology Series B: Psychological Sciences and Social Sciences, 66B*(6), 708-718.

Crivello, G. (2011). 'Becoming somebody': Youth transitions through education and migration in Peru. *Journal of Youth Studies, 14*(4), 395-411.

Dong, X., Chang, E.-S., Wong, E., & Simon, M. (2012). The perceptions, social determinants, and negative health outcomes associated with depressive symptoms among U.S. Chinese older adults. *Gerontologist, 52*(5), 650-663.

Erikson, E.H. (1968). *Identity and the life cycle.* New York: W.W. Norton & Company.

Erikson, E.H. (1980). *Identity: Youth and crisis.* New York: W.W. Norton & Company.

Fingerman, K.L., Miller, L.M., Birditt, K.S., & Zarit, S.H. (2009). Giving to the good and the needy: Parental support of grown children. *Journal of Marriage and Family, 71,* 1220-1233.

Fingerman, K.L., VanderDrift, L.E., Dotterer, A.M., Birditt, K.S., & Zarit, S.H. (2011). Support to aging parents and grown children in Black and White families. *The Gerontologist, 51*(4), 441-452.

Goins, R.T., Spencer, S.M., McGuire, L.C., Goldberg, J., Wen, Y., & Henderson, J.A. (2010). Adult caregiving among American Indians: The role of cultural factors. *The Gerontologist, 51*(3), 310-320.

Juang, L.P., & Nguyen, H.H. (2010). Ethnic identity among Chinese-American youth: The role of family obligation and community factors on ethnic engagement, clarity, and pride, *Identity: An International Journal of Theory and Research* 10: 20-38.

Kim, K., Zarit, S.H., Eggebeen, D.J., Birditt, K.S., & Fingerman, K.L. (2011). Discrepancies in reports of support exchanges between aging parents and their middle-aged children. *The Journals of Gerontology Series B: Psychological Sciences and Social Sciences, 66B*(5), 527-537.

Kim, K., Zarit, S.H., & Han, G. (2011). The structure of intergenerational exchanges of middle-aged adults with their parents and parents-in-law in Korea. Poster presented at the 64 th Annual Scientific Meeting of the Gerontological Society of America (Boston, MA).

King, V., Ledwell, M., & Pearce-Morris J. (2013). Religion and ties between adult children and their parents. *The Journals of Gerontology Series B: Psychological Sciences and Social Sciences, 68B*(5), 825-826.

Leinaweaver, J.B. (2010). Kinship paths to and from the New Europe: A unified analysis of Peruvian adoption and migration. *Journal of Latin American and Caribbean Anthropology, 16*(2), 380-400.

Lewis, J.P. (2011). Successful aging through the eyes of Alaska Native elders: What it means to be an elder in Bristol Bay, AK. *The Gerontologist, 51*(4), 540-549.

Phinney, J.S. (1992). The Multigroup Ethnic Identity Measure: A new scale for use with diverse groups. *Journal of Adolescent Research, 7,* 156-176.

Phinney, J.S., Ong, A.D., & Tanya, M. (2000). Cultural values and intergenerational value discrepancies in immigrant and non-immigrant families, *Child*

Development, 71, 528-539.

Roberts, R.E.L., & Bengtson, V.L. (1990). Is intergenerational solidarity a unidimensional construct?: A second test of a formal model. *The Journals of Gerontology: Psychological Sciences and Social Sciences, 45*, S12-S20.

Roberts, R.E.L., & Bengtson, V.L. (1996). Affective ties to parents in early adulthood and self-esteem across 20 years. *Social Psychology Quarterly, 59*, 96-106.

Silverstein, M., Gans, D., Lowenstein, A., Giarruso, R., & Bengtson, V.L. (2010). Older parent-child relationships in six developed nations: Comparisons at the intersection of affection and conflict. *Journal of Marriage and Family, 72*, 1006-1021.

Tseng, W., Hoshino, K., Hikoyeda, N., Gallagher-Thompson, D., Inoue, H., & Ventura, J. (2012). Cultural identity and intergenerational support among Latino and Asian Americans. Poster presented at the 75 th Annual Scientific Meeting of the Gerontological Society of America (San Diego, CA).

Chapter 3　Cultural Identity, Intergenerational Relationships, and Social Policies among Diverse Immigrants in Sweden

Kazumi Hoshino

INTRODUCTION

This chapter will address three issues. First, the author will examine history and demography of immigrants in Sweden and represent the Swedish mental health policies. Second, the author will analyze mental health among Asian immigrants who mainly come from China, India, and Thailand in terms of cultural identity and intergenerational relationships, by comparing mental health among immigrants from Finland, and South and East Europe as well as refugees from Middle-East and Somalia. Finally, the author will propose the policy implications of mental health for Asian immigrants from the perspectives of cultural identity and intergenerational relationships.

HISTORY, DEMOGRAPHY, AND MENTAL HEALTH POLICIES IN SWEDEN

Definition of Immigrants in Sweden

In this chapter, the author defines immigrants to Sweden as inhabitants of foreign backgrounds and their descendants, including foreign-born and children of international migrants. The population of immigrants is comprised of foreign-born persons, those who were born in Sweden to two parents born abroad, and those who were born in Sweden to one parents born abroad. Swedish immigrants includes immigrants who have Swedish citizenship, temporary and circular migrants, refugees, and adopted children who were born in other countries.

History of Immigrant in Sweden

In terms of history of immigrants, according to Hjern (2009), in the period between 1850 and 1930, 1.4 million Swedes, or about 20% of the Swedish population mostly emigrated to North America. The returnees also dominated immigration to Sweden.

During the 1930s and 1940s, the trend shifted, and the proportion of foreign-born people in the Swedish population has gradually increased. During the 1940s, it was primarily refugees from the Second World War. During the 1950s and 1960s, there was a big demand for labor from Nordic countries. Immigrants also came from Southern Europe and Turkey. At the beginning of the 1970s, the demand for labor in Swedish industry fell drastically and refugees as well as their relatives have dominated to Sweden ever since.

In the 1970s and 1980s, many refugees from the dictatorships in Latin America and the Islamic revolution in Iran settled in Sweden. During the 1990s and the first year of the 2000s, refugees have come mainly from the disintegrating former Yugoslavia and the Soviet Union as well as from civil war plagued Iraq and Somalia.

Demography of Immigrant in Sweden

With regard to recent demography, according to OECD (2012), the Swedish population reached 9.5 million in 2011, and the population of foreign-born people in Sweden was 1.4 million, 15% of the total population. Immigration to Sweden consisted of immigrants who mainly came from Finland, Poland, Denmark, and Turkey as well as refugees from Iraq, Afghanistan, the Former Yugoslavia, Iran, and Somalia. In 2011, the largest group was returning Swedish from Finland, followed by Iraq, Poland, Afghanistan, Denmark, and Somalia. The reasons of immigration to Sweden were varied such as labor migrants (21%), family reunification (20%), immigration under EU/EES rules of free movement (18%), international students (14%), and refugees (12%) in 2010 (Statistika Centralbyrau, 2012).

Mental Health Policies in Sweden

Next, the author will focus on mental health policies and laws against discrimination in Sweden to clarify the governmental basic attitudes toward immigrants, people with disabilities, and other minorities. According to the Swedish Institute (2012), the Act concerning Support and Service for Persons with Certain Functional Impairments (LSS) was enforced in 1994. It is a human-rights law designed to offer people with extensive disabilities greater opportunities to lead independent lives, and to ensure that they have equal living conditions and full participation in communities. It can offer support in the form of personal assistance in their lives, counselling, housing with special services, or assistance for parents whose children have disabilities.

In 2009, the Discrimination Act was introduced in Sweden, its general purpose being to strengthen the legal protection of the individual and to help victims of discrimination obtain redress and financial compensation. The Act combats discrimination on the grounds of gender, ethnicity, religion, disability, sexual orientation, or age, and is divided into two parts. The proactive part imposes a duty to take positive action and concerns working life, the educational system, and in other areas of society. The reactive part deals with the prohibition of discrimination in these areas. The Equality Ombudsman monitors compliance with these laws.

In 2011, the Swedish government launched a new strategy to guide its disability policy for the period leading up to 2016. The aim is to give people with disabilities a greater chance of participating in a society on the same terms as others. The special attention has been given three priority areas: The justice system; transportation; and IT. For example, as the justice system, all people should feel that the laws are reasonable, and that the justice system exists for them and ensures compliance with their legal rights. Accordingly, police authorities must analyze their operations from a disability perspective. In 2010, the Swedish Prosecution Authority initiated a project to access how it disseminates information to crime victims with disabilities and how they may absorb such information. In 2012, the Swedish National Courts Administration decided that it would develop an action plan for making Swedish courts more accessible.

MENTAL HEALTH, CULTURAL IDENTITY, AND INTERGENERATIONAL RELATIONSHIPS IN SWEDEN

Cultural Identity among Immigrants in Sweden

In this section, the author will analyze mental health among Asian immigrants to Sweden in terms of cultural identity and intergenerational relationships, by comparing mental health among immigrants as well as refugees from other parts of the world. With regard to cultural identity,

Chapter 3   Cultural Identity, Intergenerational Relationships, and Social Policies among Diverse Immigrants in Sweden   69

Wiking, Johansson, and Sundquist (2004) reported that among Iranian and Turkish men there was a threefold increased risk of poor self-reported health than Swedes, while the risk was five times higher for women in the logistic model. The Iranian and the Turkish had a higher risk of poor health than the Polish. The highest risk of the Turkish and Iranian men for poor self-reported health decreased to non-significance after the inclusion of socioeconomic status, low acculturation, and discrimination. In sum, the strong association between ethnicity and poor self-reported health may be mediated by socioeconomic status, poor acculturation, and discrimination.

From qualitative studies, Kim (2012) suggested that cultural identity among Korean immigrants continued to be mediated within social contexts in Sweden when they were involved in the process of constructing their substantive citizenship. Such dynamic processes related to legal status, memberships in communities, previous educational background, as well as work experience and then developed the heterogeneity of cultural identity. Raka (2009) also described how cultural identity had high importance among Kosovar Albanians in Sweden as they tried to understand the different cultures in the host country while they developed their ethnic communities to maintain their values and cultural practices. In addition, Raka (2009) emphasized religious identity among Kosovar Albanians who were willing to do religious activities with more time and space in the new country. Even though they were not fully practical Muslims and adjusted to the Swedish society, they stressed their religious beliefs and felt a sense of guilty when they were unable to commit to daily religious activities.

Intergenerational Relationships among Immigrants in Sweden

Next, the author will talk about intergenerational relationships among immigrants in Sweden. Malmberg and Pettersson (2007) revealed that as many as 85% of parents above retirement age had at least one adult child within a commuting distance of 50km, and that as many as 10% had an adult child living within 100 meters to the parents. However, the results did not refute previous studies that intergenerational distances were larger, and that contacts were less frequent in Sweden than most other European countries. The less wealthy and the less educated live closer by and have more access to the social capital of nearby relatives, but also that they were more tied to these relatives and to the place where they lived. Among immigrants, especially those who had recently immigrated and those coming from low-income countries, had shorter intergenerational distances as well.

On the other hand, in terms of interviews with South Asians from India, Pakistan, and Sri Lanka to Scandinavian countries such as Sweden and Denmark, Singla (2008) proposed the reinterpretation of the self and home in the immigrant families for the parental as well as the young generation. Young adults' cultural identity involved the ancestral countries and the Scandinavian welfare societies. They experienced changes in regard to parental generation and their own life understanding, as most built families and networks. They developed intergenerational relationships and attachments across the borders, in varying the extents from yearly visits to almost no visit to the country of origin. They were able to feel at home in multiple contexts. Using global technologies and microelectronic transnationalism - internet, films, and music – contributed in creating home, not only in the country of residence, but also in the country of origin and in some countries where the diaspora relations and business existed.

Mental Health among Immigrants in Sweden

In this section, the author will examine mental health among immigrants in Sweden. Hollander (2013) analyzed population-based data to clarify associations between social determinants of health and inequalities in mental health among refugees and other immigrants in Sweden. There was a significant difference in mental health between female refugees and non-refugees when adjusted for socioeconomic factors. However, refugees had a higher likelihood of poor mental health than non-refugees of the same origin. Regarding the relative risk of hospitalization due to depressive disorder following unemployment, the lowest relative risk was found among Swedish-born men and the highest among foreign-born females. Immigrants, and particularly refugees had poorer mental health than native Swedes.

However, Lindert, Schouler-Ocak, Heinz, and Priebe (2008) suggested that it was impossible to consider immigrants as a homogeneous group concerning the risk for mental illness. The literature showed that mental health differed among ethnic groups, access to psychological care facilities was influenced by the legal frame of the host country, and that mental health and consumption of care facilities were shaped by immigrants used patterns of help-seeking and by the legal frame of the host country. However, longitudinal studies are needed to describe mental health adjusting for life conditions in Sweden and other European countries to identify those factors which imply an increased risk of psychiatric disorders and influence help seeking for psychological care. In many European countries, immigrants fall outside the existing health and social services, particularly asylum seekers and underdocumented immigrants.

Cultural Identity, Intergenerational Relationships, and Mental Health

In the last part of this section, the author will focus on associations between cultural identity, intergenerational relationships, and mental health among immigrants in Sweden. As Kwak (2003) pointed out, the cultural distance between the culture of origin and that of the new country may threaten the harmony of immigrant family relations, but when the core cultural values of family embeddedness are supported by their own culture as well as their own ethnocultural social network, immigrant families can maintain healthy intergenerational relationships. Immigrant adolescents from collectivistic societies sustain these positive family relationships in part by delaying their pursuit of autonomy.

As with non-immigrant families, socioeconomic hardship in immigrant families necessitates collaboration by family members. However, unlike the former, collaboration and participation by family members in the latter are encouraged by their own ethnic culture as well. Consequently, experiences of hardships do not result in overtly adverse effects on intergenerational relationships within immigrant families.

POLICY IMPLICATIONS OF MENTAL HEALTH AMONG IMMIGRANTS IN SWEDEN

In this final section, the author will propose seven policy implications of mental health among Asian immigrants in Sweden. Hjern (2009) pointed out that few people were as dependent on Swedish law and the Swedish authorities as asylum seekers. Sweden is one of the countries in Europe that restricts the right to medical care of people without a residence permit. It is likely that these rules have mainly affected the public health of asylum

Chapter 3 Cultural Identity, Intergenerational Relationships, and Social Policies among Diverse Immigrants in Sweden 73

seekers and irregular immigrants who do not receive treatment for their illnesses and help with their disabilities. But they also affect the health of the rest of the population insofar as contagious diseases among people with limited rights to medical treatment are identified later in the course of the disease and therefore, are spread more easily.

In terms of diversity, the Swedish need to deepen understandings of diversity from the perspectives of immigrants and refugees. Torres (2001, 2003, 2006a) urged that as middle-aged Iranian immigrants suggested, there was a relationship between the cultural values that people upheld and the way they made sense of the construct of healthy aging. The migratory life course could lead to a revision of our understandings of healthy aging.

As policy issues, Hoshino (2012) suggested that health care policies needed to balance formal and informal social support programs as well as health care systems in national and local governments, by finding appropriate places for cultural diversity and universalism. Policymakers and health care professionals should develop culturally sensitive health care services and social welfare programs which correspond support needs among diverse ethnic populations.

In terms of social inclusion, Torres (2006b, 2012) pointed out that elderly immigrants were "othered" in the debate on migrants on the basis of their old age. Older people will require that we regard them as "our" elders and not just "theirs," as Swedish old-age policy has been shown to do (Machat, 2010). Hjern (2009) also suggested that discrimination might have affected mental health among immigrants.

With regard to research design, as Kwak (2003) summarized, comprehensive models of research and clinical practices for immigrants should consider associations between mental health, intergenerational relationships, and cultural identity. Immigration studies should be conducted as longitudinal surveys of ethnic subgroups among immigrants in Sweden. It is important that studies currently available in the literature are limited to immigrant group which have settled in a small number of Western individualistic countries. Considering that migration movements are increasing under globalization, more effort needs to be put into examining the characteristics of the many other migrating groups and their receiving societies.

From the worldwide perspectives, Sole-Auro and Crimmins (2008) proposed that international organizations such as European Union should have information on the area of origin of migrants and how that differs across countries in terms of analyses of the Survey of Health, Aging, and Retirement in Europe (SHARE) database which consisted 11 European countries such as Sweden, Germany, France, Switzerland, Austria, the Netherlands, Denmark, Belgium, Spain, Italy, and Greece. Future research should examine the link between health of immigrants and the place of origin. The SHARE is useful in expanding our understanding of current health issues facing Europe, and provides baseline information which policymakers can predict the impact of growing immigration on the health and social security needs of a growing and aging immigrant population.

Finally, global network and research system of mental health through lifespan development should be developed. As Hjern (2009) recommended that global migration network of physical and mental health would be needed among immigrants who have suffered severe mental illness beyond borders. In particular, refugees have experienced hardships such as violence, abuse, injury, and attacks in their home countries. Even they can access to health care in their new country, these nations may not have

Chapter 3 Cultural Identity, Intergenerational Relationships, and Social Policies among Diverse Immigrants in Sweden 75

enough information before and after immigration. Therefore, global migration network of physical and mental health should have possibilities to support immigrants beyond borders in order to minimize adversity and to promote their healthy lifespan development.

ACKNOWLEDGMENTS

This study was partly presented at the 79 the Annual Convention at the Japanese Psychological Association in Kyoto, Japan (Hoshino, 2014). The author appreciates that Dr. Winston Tseng accepted my invitation to be a presenter at the 2014 International Symposium in Japan. The author also wishes to thank Ms. Hazuki Inoue for her support as a research assistant. The study was funded by the Health Science Center (Principal Investigator: Kazumi Hoshino).

REFERENCES

Hjern, A. (2009). Migration and public health. In the National Board of Health and Welfare (Ed.) *Swedish National Public Health Report 2009*. Stockholm: The National Board of Health and Welfare.

Hollander, A.-C. (2013). Social inequalities in mental health and mortality among refugees and other immigrants to Sweden: Epidemiological studies of register data. *Global Health Action, 6,* 1-11.

Hoshino, K. (2012). Sociocultural support model for healthy aging: Perspectives from the United States, Sweden, and Japan. In A.E. Scharlach, & K. Hoshino (Eds.) *Healthy aging in sociocultural context* (pp.86-97). New York: Routledge.

Kim, O.T. (2012). *Exploring lived citizenship of Korean immigrant women in Sweden.* Lund: Lund University (unpublished master thesis).

Kwak, K. (2003). Adolescents and their parents: A review of intergenerational family relations for immigrant and non-immigrant families. *Human Development, 46,*

115-136.

Lindert, J., Schouler-Ocak, M., Heinz, A., & Priebe, S. (2008). Mental health, health care utilization of migrants in Europe. *European Psychiatry, 23*, S14-S20.

Machat, L. (2010). Bilden av "alder invandrare" I aldrepolitiken [Images of "elderly immigrants" in social policy for older people]. In S. Torres, & F. Magnusson (Eds.) *Invandrarskap, aldrevard och omsorg [Migrantship and elderly care]* (pp.55-68). Malmo: Gleerups.

Malmberg, G., & Pettersson, A. (2007). Distance to elderly parents: Analyses of Swedish register data. *Demographic Research, 17* (23), 679-704. Rostock, Germany: The Max Planck Institute for Demographic Research.

Organisation for Economic Corporation and Development (2012). *OECD migration outlook 2011.* Paris: OECD.

Raka, S.B. (2009). *Kosovar Albanian identity within migration in the Swedish society: International migration and ethnic relations.* Malmo: Malmo University (unpublished dissertation).

Singla, R. (2009). South Asians in Scandinavia: Diasporic identity processes. In A. Gari, & K. Mylonas (Eds.) *Quod Erat Demonstradum: From Herodotus' Ethnographic Journeys to Cross-Cultural Research* (pp.289-300). Athen: Pedio Books Publishing.

Sole-Auro, A., & Crimmins, E.M. (2008). Health of immigrants in European countries. *International Migration Review, 42* (4), 861-876.

Statistika Centralbyrau (2012).

Swedish Institute (2012). Facts about Sweden: Disability Policy. Retrieved July 13, 2014 from https://sweden.se/wp-content/uploads/2013/11/disability-policy-in-sweden-hight-res1.pdf

Torres, S. (2001). Understanding of successful aging in the context of migration: The case of Iranian immigrants to Sweden. *Ageing and Society, 21* (3), 333-355.

Torres, S. (2003). A preliminary empirical test of a culturally-relevant theoretical framework for the study of successful aging. *Journal of Cross-Cultural Gerontology, 18*, 73-91.

Torres, S. (2006a). Different ways of understanding the construct of successful aging: Iranian immigrants speak about what aging well means to them. *Journal of Cross-Cultural Gerontology, 21* (1-2), 1-23.

Torres, S. (2006b). Elderly immigrants in Sweden: "Otherness" under construction. *Journal of Ethnic and Migration Studies, 32* (8), 1341-1358.

Torres, S. (2012). Healthy aging among immigrants in Sweden: What we know and need to find out. In A.E. Scharlach, & K. Hoshino (Eds.) *Healthy aging in sociocultural context* (pp.62-76). New York: Routledge.

Wiking, E., Johansson, S.-E., & Sundquist, J. (2004). Ethnicity, acculturation, and self-reported health: A population-based study among immigrants from Poland, Turkey, and Iran in Sweden. *Journal of Epidemiology and Community Health, 58*, 574-582.

Part 2

International Migration and Wellness Innovation in Japan

Chapter 4 Development of the Multigroup Ethnic Identity Measure-Revised Japanese Version

Kazumi Hoshino

INTRODUCTION

International Migration and Super-Aging Societies

In a current cross-border movement, it is essential to clarify ethnic identity of younger and older populations in Japan with an appropriate psychological measure, even though historically the country has been considered a homogenous society. This is the first study to develop the Multigroup Ethnic Identity Measure-Revised (MEIM-R) Japanese version and to establish reliability and validity of the scale among younger and older adults in Japan.

In global aging societies with growing aging populations, lower fertility rates, declining labor force, and increasing numbers of immigrants, psychological studies on ethnic identity are the most important areas of interdisciplinary research to support human development among younger and older adults of native-born nationals as well as immigrants. Comparing the population structure in the United States and Japan (World Bank, 2012), the percentage of the young population (0-14 years old) was 20%; that of the working-age population (15-64 years old) was 67%; and that of the elderly population (65 years and older) was 13% in the United States. These percentages were 14%, 63%, and 23% in Japan, respectively. In 2007-2011,

82   Part 2   International Migration and Wellness Innovation in Japan

net migration was 4,954,924 in the United States and 270,000 in Japan.

The current challenges in the United States and Japan are how each generation can promote lifespan development mutually in the midst of considerable family diversity (Fingerman, Miller, Birditt, & Zarit, 2009; Kim, Zarit, Eggebeen, Birditt, & Fingerman, 2011; Fingerman, VanderDrift, Dotterer, Birditt, & Zarit, 2011), and how they can actualize social integration in unprecedented multicultural and multigenerational communities (Hoshino, 2012a). Reflecting the importance of socioeconomic status, international students, migrant workers, and immigrants are more vulnerable to societal, social, and familial changes than native-born nationals. On the other hand, Japanese nationals may examine their ethnic identity and consider how they can support immigrants with openness to diversity. Such psychological studies on ethnic identity are particularly vital to these nations, as well as other countries that have similar issues.

Ethnic Identity and Demographic Changes in Japan

Japan is considered an industrialized democratic country that has developed a strong attachment to ethnic identity and has reinforced the nation's ethnic homogeneity (Kalicki, 2009). The unique quality of "Japaneseness" is described that "the Japanese constitute a culturally and socially homogenous racial entity, whose essence is virtually unchanged from prehistorical times down to the present day," which differentiates the Japanese people from other people (Dale, 1986, p.1). Also, the Japanese national character is viewed as having an "ethnocentric emphasis on the nation as the preeminent collective identity of the people," which, as a societal force, has shaped the way Japanese regard themselves (Kowner, 1999, p.250).

Chapter 4　Development of the Multigroup Ethnic Identity Measure-Revised Japanese Version　　83

However, as the author mentioned earlier, unprecedented demographic changes, including higher life expectancy, lower fertility rates, and declining working-age populations have occurred for a few decades in Japan. The shortages of labor force have led to accepting immigrants and migrant workers. Also, since Japanese youth are reluctant to engage in manual labor and professional caregiving jobs, the entry of unskilled migrant workers of the Japanese descendants and caregivers from the Philippines and Indonesia was facilitated by the amendments of the Immigration Control and Refugee Recognition Acts since 1990 (Mackie, 2010). In addition, international marriage is regarded as a form of labor migration, in which the women who immigrate as wives of Japanese men become domestic caregivers (Mackie, 1998, 2010; Piquero-Ballescas, 2009). Consequently, one in every 30 babies was born from at least one foreign partner, and nearly 6.5% of the total marriages were international (McNeil et al., 2009).

Under such transitions, researchers should clarify dynamic processes how Japanese younger and older adults, who accurately reflect demographic changes, have formed ethnic identity and how ethnic identity is created through interactions between younger and older generations. As ethnic identity studies have not focused on Japanese nationals, in particular older adults, we need to examine ethnic identity among Japanese younger adults as well as older adults and to develop appropriate psychological measures of ethnic identity in Japanese. Historical, social, and cultural events may have affected ethnic identity throughout lifespan development. Specifically, older adults have experienced World War Two and postwar economic growth and recessions. Since older adults have faced societal shifts before and after the War, the author needs to examine ethnic identity among older adults along

84   Part 2   International Migration and Wellness Innovation in Japan

with younger adults.

Concepts of Ethnic Identity

Ethnic identity is defined as an aspect of a person's social identity, "that part of an individual's self-concept which derives from [his/her] knowledge of [his/her] membership in a social group (or groups) together with the value and emotional significance attached to that membership"(Tajfel, 1981, p.255). On the other hand, cultural identity is defined as a part of identity in which a person feels the membership he/she belongs to cultural groups not only of ethnicity but also of other social/cultural groups such as gender, sexual orientation, deaf, disability, and so forth (Banks, 2006). Therefore, the concept of cultural identity is broader than that of ethnic identity, and includes ethnic identity.

Erikson (1968, 1980) regarded ethnic identity as a part of identity formation in ethnicity. "The growing child must derive a vitalizing sense of reality from the awareness that his individual ways of mastering experience (his ego synthesis) is a successful variant of a group identity, and is in accord with its space-time and life span" (Erikson, 1980, p.21). Erikson (1980) also remarked that youth became intolerant in their exclusion of others who were different in cultural background as the signs of an in-grouper or out-grouper, in which such intolerance might be a necessary defense against a sense of identity loss.

Based on Erikson's work on psychosocial development, Marcia (1966, 1980) proposed a concept of identity status that involved exploration of identity and commitment to identity domains and classified individuals into four developmental statuses: Achievement; Foreclosure; Moratorium; and Diffusion. Marcia (2010) also suggested that identity status shifts

Chapter 4   Development of the Multigroup Ethnic Identity Measure-Revised Japanese Version   85

throughout lifespan development, and reconstruction processes included the moratorium-achievement-moratorium-achievement (MAMA) cycles. Once identity status is established in adolescence, the MAMA cycle is anticipated to reoccur a minimum of three cycles, corresponding to young adulthood, adulthood, and late life. Like ego identity, ethnic identity is developed throughout life (Ong, Fuller-Rowell, & Phinney, 2010), even after the major developmental changes are assumed to occur in adolescence and young adulthood, and a stable sense of ethnic identity is achieved or continues to be explored in adulthood (Phinney & Ong, 2007).

The Multigroup Ethnic Identity Measure (MEIM)

According to Phinney (1990, 1992), psychological measures of ethnic identity have focused on different ethnic groups such as African Americans (Cross, 1978), Hispanics (Arce, 1981), Asians (Makabe, 1979), and Europeans (Rosenthal & Hrynevich, 1985). Although these scales deal with specific aspects that closely relate to each ethnic group including language, religious affiliation and activities, and cultural traditions and practices, ethnic identity scales are needed to gain commonalities of ethnic identity beyond differences of individual groups. Phinney (1992) developed the Multigroup Ethnic Identity Measure (MEIM) for diverse ethnic groups. The MEIM consisted of 14 items assessing ethnic identity and six items assessing other-group orientation. An exploratory factor analysis of the 14-item MEIM revealed three components of ethnic identity: Ethnic Affirmation and Belonging (seven items); Ethnic Identity Achievement (five items); and Ethnic Behaviors (two items). With regard to construct validity, the MEIM for minorities was significant and positively correlated to self-esteem among the high school and the college students. For European Americans, the

MEIM was not related to self-esteem among the college students, while it was significant and positively correlated to self-esteem among the high school students. To organize both subscales as one whole measure of ethnic identity, Phinney (1992) decided that the whole scale had a two-factor structure: the 14-item MEIM; and the Other-group orientation scale.

Next, Roberts, Phinney, Masse, Chen, Roberts, and Romeo (1999) conducted exploratory and confirmatory factor analyses and found that a two-factor structure best fitted the data: Affirmation, Belonging, and Commitment (seven items); and Exploration (five items). Roberts et al. (1999) deleted two items, which were negatively worded and did not fit the model. The 12- item MEIM was significant and positively correlated to self-esteem, mastery, coping strategies, and optimism, although it was significant and negatively correlated to depression and loneliness.

Reliability and validity of the MEIM have been widely examined (Ponterotto & Mallinckrodt, 2007; Ponterotto & Park-Taylor, 2007). Gaines et al. (2010) argued whether the 14-item MEIM holds a single dimensional measure or multiple dimensional measures, and exploratory and confirmatory analyses revealed a three-factor structure: the Behavioral Component; the Cognitive Component; and the Affective Component. However, the sample was small and contained specific ethnic groups (Ong, Fuller-Rowell, & Phinney, 2010).

In Japan, Uematsu (2010) translated the 14-item MEIM (Phinney, 1992) from English into Japanese, and an exploratory factor analysis found a two-factor structure for native-born Japanese in Japan and Japanese students living in the United States: Exploration; and Affirmation, Belonging, and Commitment. However, Uematsu (2010) did not report how the translation was conducted, including whether back-translation was used. Also, a factor analysis was conducted for the whole group, although international students had significantly higher scores on these subscales than native-born nationals. In addition, the scale included only 10 of the 14 items, though the outcome was similar to other studies, with factors of Exploration (six items) and Affirmation, Belonging, and Commitment (four items). Four items were deleted due to the exclusion of items with factor loadings less than .50 and/or with modest factor loadings of more than .30 on two scales.

Sugioka and Kodama (2005) translated the 12-item MEIM (Roberts et al., 1999) from English into Japanese, and then from Japanese into Portuguese, each with a back translation by a bilingual translator. The Portuguese version was not directly translated from English to Portuguese, and such development procedures were questioned on translation accuracy. Also, the Portuguese version included 24 items because they prepared two items for each question. One item asked about Japanese ethnic identity, and the other item asked about Brazilian ethnic identity. As a result, each 12-item MEIM had one factor and did not examine a two or more-factor structure by confirmatory and exploratory factor analyses.

Therefore, further work is needed that uses appropriate procedures of translation and that clarifies the factor structure. Moreover, this work should be done using the MEIM-R, which has advantages over the MEIM, but has not been translated for use in Japan. Further, given Marcia's model of lifelong identity development, comparative studies between younger and older generations need to be conducted to clarify ethnic identity. Although ethnic identity development is assumed across lifespan, there are few studies to examine different generations, in particular elderly populations.

The Multigroup Ethnic Identity Measure-Revised (MEIM-R)

In consideration of the previous studies, a remaining issue of the MEIM is the debate about whether the scale consists of a single-factor structure or a two- or more-factor structure, although Exploration and Commitment are essential for assessing ethnic identity among diverse ethnic groups. Phinney and Ong (2007) presented the Multigroup Ethnic Identity Measure-Revised (MEIM-R). A confirmatory factor analysis for 241 university students of diverse ethnic groups found the best model was a two-factor structure: Exploration (three items); and Commitment (three items). These subscales corresponded to the typology of identity status (Marcia, 1980). Yoon (2011) also indicated associations between the MEIM-R and the Ethnic Identity Scale (Umana-Taylor, Yazedjian, & Bamaca-Gomez, 2004) and demonstrated theoretical evidence in terms of data analyses in which subscales of the MEIM-R were consistent with identity status. Thus, reliability and validity of the MEIM-R were further supported.

The strengths of the MEIM-R are to be tested by confirmatory and exploratory factor analyses in which the former clarified the goodness-of-fit of nested alternative models systematically, and the latter could be descriptive for the testing of model contrasts. Also, as the subscales of the MEIM-R covers the concepts of exploration and commitment that derive from identity status theory (Marcia, 1980), these scales are comparable and can be used separately as well. In addition, the MEIM-R includes only six items and may lead to usability as it can be easily combined with additional measures for other aspects of ethnic identity of specifically targeted ethnic groups and other variables, depending on researchers' study aims.

Present Study

In sum, there are few intergenerational comparative studies of ethnic identity between younger and older adults, and previous work on ethnic identity has mainly focused on youth (Ong, Fuller-Rowell, & Phinney, 2010). Ethnic identity research is particularly important to conduct among different generations, specifically among younger and older adults that reflect current demographic changes of declining working-age population and increasing elderly population in Japan. In addition, the MEIM-R is regarded as having a stable two-factor structure according to theoretical basis and empirical data analyses (Yoon, 2011). Furthermore, the MEIM-R is considered as having higher usability for younger and older adults when the author implement a questionnaire that consists of other physical, social, and psychological measures. In particular, a welcome development of the Japanese version would be an appropriate factor analysis to conduct comparative studies between younger and older generations.

The present study examines ethnic identity among Japanese younger and older adults. Although considered ethnically homogeneous, recently Japan has been noticing the importance of diversity and trying to accept immigrants. Given this transition, ethnic identity should be evaluated with an appropriate psychological measure. The goal of this study is to develop the Multigroup Ethnic Identity Measure-Revised (MEIM-R) Japanese version with appropriate indicators of reliability and validity.

This study expects that the MEIM-R Japanese version will have a two-factor structure: Exploration; and Commitment, which is similar to the original work by Phinney & Ong (2007). The author also anticipates that the subscales each will have higher Cronbach's alpha values which support reliability of the MEIM-R Japanese version. In addition, the present study

90   Part 2   International Migration and Wellness Innovation in Japan

has expectations that the subscales will significantly correlate to cultural identity scale in order to confirm the validity of the MEIM-R Japanese version. To select an appropriate measure of cultural identity, the Scale to Measure Banks' Cultural Identity (SBCI: Hoshino, Nakayama, Iwasa, & Zarit, 2010) is focused. This is because the theory represents strengths as the development of cultural identity with a global perspective, and the SBCI can effectively evaluate cultural identity, which consists of a three factor structure: From Multiculturalism to Globalism; From Cultural Encapsulation to Biculturalism; and From Cultural Psychological Captivity to Cultural Identity Clarification. The author anticipates that Exploration and Commitment each will significantly relate to the subscales of the SBCI. The author also expects that Exploration will have higher correlation to the subscales of the SBCI than Commitment will do. Because higher Exploration to ethnic identity may further relate to the development of cultural identity with a global perspective, while Commitment to ethnic identity may partly relate to that of cultural identity in this homogenous country.

METHODS

Participants

The sample consisted of 443 participants including 203 Japanese younger adults (114 men, 89 women) and 240 Japanese older adults (130 men, 110 women) who lived independently in central region of Japan. The mean age of younger adults was 19.28 years old (SD=1.04), and that of older adults was 69.25 years old (SD=4.78). At one university, 235 younger adults answered a questionnaire in their classes, if they agreed to participate in an

Chapter 4   Development of the Multigroup Ethnic Identity Measure-Revised Japanese Version   91

international research project. At the Senior Citizen College, 525 older adults were invited during classes they attended to participate in the project, and 271 older adults returned questionnaires by mail. Of these, the questionnaires of 32 younger adults and 31 older adults were excluded from data because of more than one-third missing items on each one scale. The respondent rate among younger adults was 86.38%, the rate among older adults was 45.71%, and the total was 58.29%. The College was a lifelong learning institute, and all participants were community-dwelling older adults.

The Institutional Review Board of the Senior Citizen College approved this study. The participants signed the informed consent form upon their agreement. The project team kept questionnaires confidential and coded them with participants' ID numbers in order to exclude individual identifying information from data.

Measures

A self-reported questionnaire consisted of the Japanese versions of the MEIM-R, the Scale to Measure Banks's Cultural Identity (SBCI: Hoshino et al., 2010), questions about the participants' social characteristics, and other measures. However, this chapter focused on only the MEIM-R, the SBCI, and questions concerning the participants' social characteristics, as the author examined other measures in chapter 5.

Ethnic Identity: Phinney (1992) developed the Multigroup Ethnic Identity Measure (MEIM: 20 items), and Phinney and Ong (2007) presented the Multigroup Ethnic Identity Measure-Revised (MEIM-R: six items). The MEIM-R had a two-factor structure: Exploration; and Commitment. The

92   Part 2 International Migration and Wellness Innovation in Japan

reliability was supported by higher Cronbach's alpha values for each subscale, and validity of the scale was confirmed due to the correspondence between the subscales and identity status typology (Marcia, 1966, 1980). Ratings of the Japanese version were made on a five-point scale from 1 (strongly disagree) to 5 (strongly agree).

In the development process of the Japanese version, first a Japanese/English bilingual researcher of psychology translated the original MEIM and MEIM-R from English into Japanese. Another Japanese/English bilingual researcher independently back-translated it. Second, the two researchers examined translation accuracy so that the Japanese version could appropriately convey the concept of ethnic identity and the original MEIM and MEIM-R in consideration of commonalities and differences of sociocultural contexts between the United States and Japan. Third, Professors Jean S. Phinney and Anthony D. Ong allowed the author to use the translated versions as Japanese versions of the MEIM and MEIM-R.

Cultural Identity: The Scale to Measure Banks's Cultural Identity (SBCI: Hoshino et al., 2010) was used to examine validity of the MEIM-R Japanese version. The SBCI consists of a three-factor structure: From Multiculturalism to Globalism (11 items); From Cultural Encapsulation to Biculturalism (seven items); and From Cultural Psychological Captivity to Cultural Identity Clarification (four items). Higher Cronbach's alpha values supported reliability of the scale, and construct validity was confirmed by significant correlations to the relevant scales and correspondence to the Cultural Identity Theory (Banks, 1976, 2006). Items were rated on a five-point scale from 1 (strongly disagree) to 5 (strongly agree). Professor James Banks allowed the author to use the SBCI which evaluates cultural identity

Chapter 4   Development of the Multigroup Ethnic Identity Measure-Revised Japanese Version   93

based on his theory.

Social Characteristics: The participants rated their social characteristics as follows. Marital status on a scale ranging from 1 (married), 2 (never married), 3 (widowed), and 4 (divorced); current job status on a scale ranging from 1 (unemployed), 2 (full-time job), and 3 (part-time job); living arrangement on a scale ranging from 1 (living alone), and 2 (living with families/others); housing on a scale ranging from 1 (their own home), and 2 (support apartment). They also answered questions about their age, gender, numbers of children and grandchildren, years of education and of past job careers.

The author coded gender as 1 (women), 0 (men); marital status as 1 (married), 0 (not married); current job status as 1 (full-time/part-time job), 0 (unemployment); living arrangement as 1 (living with families/others), 0 (living alone); housing as 1 (living in support apartment), 0 (living in their home); and age, each year of education and past job careers, and the numbers of children and of grandchildren.

Data Analysis

The present study used the IBM SPSS Version 21 for an exploratory factor analysis of the MEIM-R Japanese version to clarify a factor structure. The author also calculated Cronbach's alpha values to confirm reliability of the scale and correlations between the MEIM-R Japanese version and the SBCI to assure validity of the scale.

Table 4-1 The Participants' Social Characteristics

Social Characteristics	Younger Adults (N=203)		Older Adults (N=240)	
	M (SD)	Proportion (%)	M (SD)	Proportion (%)
Age	19.28 (1.04)		69.25 (4.78)	
Gender				
Men		114 (56.2%)		130 (54.2%)
Women		89 (43.8%)		110 (45.8%)
Marital Status				
Married		4 (2.0%)		187 (77.9%)
Never Married		199 (98.0%)		3 (1.3%)
Widowed		0 (0%)		37 (15.4%)
Divorced		0 (0%)		13 (5.4%)
Children				
Yes		0 (0%)		226 (94.2%)
No		203 (100%)		14 (5.8%)
The Number of Children	0 (0)		2.09 (0.86)	
Grandchildren				
Yes		0 (0%)		182 (75.8%)
No		203 (100%)		58 (24.2%)
The Number of Grandchildren	0 (0)		2.26 (1.82)	
Years of Education	12.73 (1.68)		13.23 (2.69)	
Years of Job Careers	0.09 (0.78)		31.71 (16.71)	
Current Job				
Unemployed		119 (58.6%)		206 (85.8%)
Full Time Job		2 (1.0%)		9 (3.8%)
Part Time Job		73 (36.0%)		25 (10.4%)
No answer		9 (4.4%)		0 (0%)
Living Arrangement				
Living Alone		122 (60.1%)		31 (12.9%)
Living with Families/Others		77 (37.9%)		208 (86.7%)
No answer		4 (2.0%)		1 (0.4%)
Housing				
Living in Their Own Home		158 (77.8%)		237 (98.8%)
Support Apartment		2 (1.0%)		3 (1.3%)
No answer		43 (21.2%)		0 (0%)

RESULTS

Participants' Social Characteristics

As the participants' social characteristics show (Table 4-1), married participants were 2.0 % among younger adults and 77.9 % among older adults. The mean of their education years was 12.73 years (SD=1.68) among younger adults and 13.23 years (SD=2.69) among older adults. The mean of their past job careers was 0.9 years (SD=0.78) among younger adults and 31.71 years (SD=16.71) among older adults. 58.6% of younger adults and 85.8% of older adults were currently unemployed. 60.1% of younger adults and 12.9% of older adults lived alone.

Factor Analysis of the MEIM-R Japanese Version

First, an exploratory factor analysis was performed for younger adults and for older adults separately and found a similar two-factor structure to Phinney and Ong (2007). Second, the author conducted an exploratory factor analysis for the whole sample and confirmed the same factor structure that Phinney and Ong (2007) had reported. As Table 4-2 shows, the first factor was named as Exploration, and the second was named as Commitment. Items of Exploration in order of higher factor loadings were "4. I have often done things that will help me understand my ethnic background better," "5. I have often talked to other people in order to learn more about my ethnic group," "1. I have spent time trying to find out more about my ethnic group, such as its history, traditions, and customs," and "3. I understand pretty well what my ethnic group membership means to me." Items of Commitment were "2. I have a strong sense of belonging to my own ethnic group," and "6. I feel a strong attachment towards my own

96   Part 2   International Migration and Wellness Innovation in Japan

Table 4-2 Principal Components Factor Analysis of the MEIM-R Japanese Version

Items / Factor Loadings	F 1	F 2	M	(SD)
Factor 1: Exploration				
4. I have often done things that will help me understand my ethnic background better.	**.957**	-.077	2.91	(1.01)
5. I have often talked to other people in order to learn more about my ethnic group.	**.792**	.030	2.60	(1.10)
1. I have spent time trying to find out more about my ethnic group, such as its history, traditions, and customs.	**.715**	.098	3.21	
3. I understand pretty well what my ethnic group membership means to me.	**.589**	.264	2.97	(1.05)
Factor 2: Commitment				
2. I have a strong sense of belonging to my own ethnic group.	.042	**.783**	3.71	(0.98)
6. I feel a strong attachment towards my own ethnic group.	.013	**.679**	3.79	(0.97)

Note: The MEIM-R=The Multigroup Ethnic Identity Measure-Revised.

ethnic group."

The one difference in the factor structure of the original MEIM-R was item 3 that belonged to Exploration in the Japanese version because of the higher factor loading, although item 3 was put into Commitment in the MEIM-R original scale (Phinney & Ong, 2007). Therefore, the Japanese version consisted of a two-factor structure: Exploration (four items); and Commitment (two items). As a result of t-test, there was no significant difference in each mean of subscales from each item between younger and older adults, although that of older adults was slightly higher than that of younger adults.

Chapter 4   Development of the Multigroup Ethnic Identity Measure-Revised Japanese Version   97

Table 4-3 Correlations between the MEIM-R and the SBCI

	The SBCI: From Multiculturalism to Globalism	From Cultural Encapsulation to Biculturalism	From Cultural Psychological Captivity to Cultural Identity Clarification
The MEIM-R: Exploration	.60***	.44***	.60***
Commitment	.33***	.30***	.44***

Note: The MEIM-R=The Multigroup Ethnic Identity Measure-Revised; The SBCI=The Scale to Measure Banks's Cultural Identity.
* $p < .05$; ** $p < .01$; *** $p < .001$.

Cronbach's Alpha Values and Correlations between the MEIM-R and the SBCI

To confirm internal consistency of the scale, Cronbach's coefficient alpha was calculated. Exploration was alpha=.89, and Commitment was alpha=.72. As Table 4-3 shows, correlations of each subscale between the MEIM-R and the SBCI were significant. Each correlation between Exploration and the subscales of the SBCI were higher than each correlation between Commitment and those of the SBCI.

DISCUSSION

Factor Structure of the MEIM-R Japanese Version

An exploratory factor analysis of the MEIM-R revealed a two-factor structure that had been reported by Phinney and Ong (2007): Exploration; and Commitment. The only difference is that item 3 yielded to Exploration in the Japanese version, while item 3 belonged to Commitment in the original scale. The Japanese version holds a two-factor structure including Exploration (four items) and Commitment (two items). Although items 2 and 6 contain a strong sense of belonging and a strong attachment to his/her ethnic group, item 3 "I understand pretty well what my ethnic group membership means to me" does not express such solid attitudes toward the participant's ethnic group. Since Japan has been historically regarded as an extremely homogeneous society, native-born nationals may seldom consider who he/she is as Japanese. Therefore, the content of item 3 concerning understanding of what Japanese means to him/her was not viewed as Commitment by this sample of younger and older adults in Japan and yielded to Exploration in this study. Also, there was no significant difference of each mean per item, although that of older adults was slightly higher than that of younger adults. This is because older adults have been aware of ethnic identity more clearly than younger adults in face of historical events such as World War Two and postwar economic growth and recession. However, such differences were not statistically significant as the Japanese may not have many opportunities to communicate with immigrants in their daily life.

Uematsu (2010) implemented an explanatory factor analysis of the 14-item MEIM and found a two-factor structure among Japanese students living in Japan and the United States. However, the translation and back translation procedures were not indicated, and the scale consisted of only 10 items since four items were excluded due to factor loadings. In addition, Uematsu (2010) did not conduct the MEIM-R for other age groups. In contrast, the present study can for the first time, demonstrate the MEIM-R Japanese version with translation accuracy and appropriate factor analysis in which the sample is composed of younger and older adults.

Reliability and Validity of the MEIM-R Japanese Version

Alpha values of the present study were that Exploration was Cronbach's coefficient alpha=.89, and Commitment was alpha=.72. Phinney and Ong (2007) reported that Exploration was alpha=.76, and Commitment was alpha=.78. Yoon (2011) also indicated that alpha =.84 was for Exploration, and alpha =.91 was for Commitment. Thus, as the author anticipated, reliability of the MEIM-R Japanese version was confirmed.

In terms of validity of the scale, the subscales of the MEIM-R and the SBCI each were significantly related. Also, each correlation between Exploration and the subscales of the SBCI were higher than each correlation between Commitment and those of the SBCI. Such outcomes supported the author's expectations of relationships between Exploration, Commitment, and the SBCI. Younger and older generations who showed higher Commitment to ethnic identity had lower correlations to cultural identity than those who showed higher Exploration to ethnic identity. Because younger and older adults who have deeply explored ethnic identity tend to indicate a prospective possibility of the higher development of cultural identity, while those who have extremely committed to ethnic identity may not develop cultural identity furthermore. Specifically, Exploration and the higher stages of cultural identity (i.e., From Multiculturalism to Globalism) had a strong correlation, and also Commitment and the lower stages of cultural identity (i.e., From Cultural Psychological Captivity to Cultural Identity Clarification) had a moderate correlation. However, the author should continue to examine the detailed relationships between each subscale of the MEIM-R and the SBCI since Exploration and the lower stages of cultural identity (i.e., From Cultural Psychological Captivity to Cultural Identity Clarification) showed a strong correlation as well. In sum, Japan has reinforced the nation's ethnic homogeneity (Kalicki, 2009), and Japanese nationals constitute a culturally and socially homogenous racial entity (Dale, 1986). Under such sociocultural contexts, it is important for this sample to understand the challenges of considering ethnic identity in this homogenous nation. Also, it is presumed that citizens may have difficulties of cultural identity development with a global perspective in Japan.

With regard to conceptual relationships, Exploration and Commitment were consistent with the concepts of exploration and commitment that are derived from empirical studies of identity status (Marcia, 1966, 1980). Yoon (2011) supported theoretical and empirical evidence between the MEIM-R and identity status (Marcia, 1966, 1980). According to Marcia's theory that exploration and commitment are two components, Yoon (2011) tested a four-cluster solution and revealed that the four groups of the MEIM-R corresponded to the four statuses of identity typology: Achievement; Foreclose; Moratorium; and Diffusion. Hence, reflecting these significant correlations between the MEIM-R and the SBCI and theoretical as well as empirical evidence (Erikson, 1968, 1980; Marcia, 1966, 1980; Phinney, 1992; Phinney & Ong, 2007; Yoon, 2011), construct validity of the MEIM-R Japanese version was also established in this study.

Immigrants in Japan

Immigrants in Japan have been facing challenges of acculturation, and societal support to immigrants should be examined at each level of national, regional and local governments, and among health care professionals (Hoshino, 2012b). Tanibuchi (2009) also suggested social support programs for immigrants of multiple generations in schools, work places, and

Chapter 4   Development of the Multigroup Ethnic Identity Measure-Revised Japanese Version   101

communities in order to promote language and cultural access to education, employment, and social participation. These studies indicate that culturally and linguistically sensitive support needs to be considered in communication with immigrants in Japan.

Kim (2011) identified factors of ethnic identity among Korean Japanese living in Japan. Korean language proficiency and Korean civic engagement were significant and positively associated with the emotional component of ethnic identity. Korean language proficiency, Korean cultural practices, and Korean civic engagement were significant and positively associated with the belonging of ethnic identity. Korean language proficiency and Korean civic engagement were significant and positively associated with the cultural understanding of ethnic identity, while gender (male) was significant and negatively associated with it. However, the ethnic identity scale which Kim (2011) developed from the MEIM did not examine reliability and validity. Future research needs to use appropriate psychological measures of ethnic identity in order to plan culturally sensitive social and health programs in their communities and to clarify trajectories between ethnic identity, cultural practices, and ethnic community activities.

Moon and Mikami (2009) examined factors that were associated with falls among older Japanese and older Korean Japanese. The significant factors were tendencies of withdrawal and taking hypnotics among Japanese, and decreased Activities of Daily Living (ADL) and visual acuity, higher prevalence of diabetes mellitus, stroke, osteoarthritis, and lower subjective well-being among Korean Japanese. There were differences in their health practices, ethnic customs, and diet preferences between two groups, and these factors influenced on falls. Prospective research should identify interactions between ethnic identity and physical and psychological

102　　Part 2　International Migration and Wellness Innovation in Japan

well-being among older Japanese, Korean Japanese, and Korean nationals.

Japanese Immigrants in the United States

Since Japan is a homogenous nation, Japanese nationals may not have many opportunities to think about ethnic identity in their daily life. Rather, in the case of going to abroad, they encounter different cultures and meditate on how they ethnically live. Iwamasa and Iwasaki (2011) analyzed qualitative data from focus groups of older Japanese Americans and selected dimensions of successful aging. Although the overall sample was fairly acculturated, older Japanese Americans maintained group harmony and focused on others more clearly than individualism and independence. Depending on their acculturation level, older Japanese Americans participated in ethnic social activities. A Japanese traditional style of inter-relationships, which engages in more ethnically expected social roles and belonging to society, was an essential element of successful aging among less acculturated older Japanese Americans.

　　On the other hand, Moriizumi (2011) described ethnic identity negotiations among Japanese younger adults who married with American men and lived in the United States. They faced negative attitudes towards the international marriages from their families and communities in Japan and experienced discrimination in the United States. Particularly, in their child rearing processes they negotiated the salience of ethnic identities and managed dialectical tensions of their children's possible identities within interracial families. Thus, Japanese who lived in the United States have convinced ethnic identity in historical contexts and racial ideologies in the United States and Japan. These findings suggest that Japanese nationals are more sensitive to ethnic identity in the United States than in Japan. As a

Chapter 4 Development of the Multigroup Ethnic Identity Measure-Revised Japanese Version   103

minority, they have to struggle with how they ethnically relate to others and communities in different social and cultural contexts. Future research is expected to compile a model of ethnic identity among Japanese nationals in Japan and overseas countries as well as immigrants in Japan.

Limitations and Future Directions

The present study has several limitations. First, the sample is not nationally representative, as older adults were healthy and belonged to a lifelong learning institute, and younger adults were university students in central region of Japan. Second, ethnic identity among adults may be identified in order to determine lifespan development processes of ethnic identity more accurately. Third, ethnic identity of immigrants in Japan should be clarified, as these groups are minorities and may face challenges of acculturation and social exclusion. Comparative studies need to be conducted for Japanese nationals as well as immigrants from adolescence to later life. In addition, future research should identify predictors of ethnic identity and clarify how international experiences and global educational programs in overseas countries, and communications with immigrants in Japan shape ethnic identity through lifespan development by using this scale. However, the present study can contribute to development of the MEIM-R Japanese version and to establish the reliability and validity of the scale in Japan, which is historically considered a homogeneous country and needs to consider diversity in an unprecedented international migration movement.

CONCLUSION

This study first developed the MEIM-R Japanese version of the same two-factor structure that Phinney and Ong (2007) had originally reported. The only difference is that item 3 belonged to Exploration, although Phinney and Ong (2007) categorized it as Commitment. As reliability and validity of the scale were confirmed, the MEIM-R Japanese version is applicable to younger and older adults in Japan. As a future direction, predictors of ethnic identity need to be identified among Japanese nationals in Japan and overseas countries as well as immigrants in Japan, drawing from a population-based data of youth, adults, and older generations.

ACKNOWLEDGMENTS

This study was partly presented at the 63rd Annual Scientific Meeting of the Gerontological Society of America in New Orleans, LA (Hoshino et al., 2010) and the 74th Annual Convention of the Japanese Psychological Association in Osaka (Nakayama & Hoshino, 2010). The author wishes to thank Professors Jean S. Phinney and Anthony D. Ong for permitting the author to use the Japanese version of the MEIM-R. The author also appreciates the Editorial Committee of the Central Japanese (Tokai) Journal of Psychology for their permission of reprinting the paper for this book. Moreover, the author would like to express gratitude to Dr. Steven H. Zarit, the participants at the Senior Citizen College and research assistants, in particular Mr. Makoto Nakayama and Ms. Hiromi Kitagawa. This study was supported by the Grant-In-Aid for Scientific Research of the Japan Society for the Promotion of Science to Kazumi Hoshino.

REFERENCES

Arce, C. (1981). A reconsideration of Chicano culture and identity. *Daedalus, 110,*

Chapter 4   Development of the Multigroup Ethnic Identity Measure-Revised Japanese Version   105

177-192.

Banks, J. (1976). The emerging stages of ethnicity: Implications for staff development. *Educational Leadership, 34*(3), 190-193.

Banks, J. (2006). *Cultural diversity and education: Foundations, curriculum, and teaching (5 th ed.)*. Boston: Pearson Education.

Cross, W. (1978). The Thomas and Cross models of psychological nigrescence: A literature review. *Journal of Black Psychology, 4*, 13-31.

Dale, P. (1986). *The myth of Japanese uniqueness*. New York: St. Martin's Press.

Erikson, E.H. (1968). *Identity: Youth and crisis*. New York: W. W. Norton & Company.

Erikson, E.H. (1980). *Identity and the life cycle*. New York: W. W. Norton & Company.

Fingerman, K.L., Miller, L.M., Birditt, K.S., & Zarit, S.H. (2009). Giving to the good and the needy: Parental support of grown children. *Journal of Marriage and Family, 71*, 1220-1233.

Fingerman, K.L., VanderDrift, L.E., Dotterer, A.M., Birditt, K.S., & Zarit, S.H. (2011). Support to aging parents and grown children in Black and White families. *The Gerontologist, 51*(4), 441-452.

Gaines, S.O., Bunce, D. Jr., Robertson, T., Wright, B., Heer, D., Lidder, A., Mann, A., & Minhas, S. (2010). Evaluating the psychometric properties of the Multigroup Ethnic Identity Measure (MEIM) within the United Kingdom. *Identity: An International Journal of Theory and Research, 10*(1), 1-19.

Hoshino, K. (2012a). Sociocultural support model for healthy aging for older immigrants: Perspectives from the United States, Sweden, and Japan. In A.E. Scharlach, & K. Hoshino (Eds.) *Healthy aging in sociocultural context* (pp.85-96). New York: Routledge.

Hoshino, K. (2012b). Healthy aging among older immigrants in Japan. In A.E. Scharlach, & K. Hoshino (Eds.) *Healthy aging in sociocultural context* (pp.72-81). New York: Routledge.

Hoshino, K., Nakayama, M., Iwasa, H., & Zarit, S.H. (2010). Multicultural educational intervention for older adults in Japan. Poster presented at the 63rd Annual Scientific Meeting of the Gerontological Society of America (New Orleans, LA).

Iwamasa, G.Y., & Iwasaki, M. (2011). A new multidimensional model of successful aging: Perceptions of Japanese American older adults. *Journal of Cross-Cultural Gerontology, 26,* 261-278.

Kalicki, K. (2009). Ethnic nationalism and political community: The overseas suffrage debates in Japan and South Korea. *Asian Studies Review, 33,* 175-195.

Kim, K., Zarit, S.H., Eggebeen, D.J., Birditt, K.S., & Fingerman, K.L. (2011). Discrepancies in reports of support exchanges between aging parents and their middle-aged children. *The Journals of Gerontology Series B: Psychological Sciences and Social Sciences, 66B*(5), 527-537.

Kim, M. (2011). Korean mass-media communication and ethnic identity among Korean Japanese. Paper presented at the Annual Scientific Meeting of the Japanese Mass-Media Communication Association (Tokyo, Japan).

Kowner, R. (1999). Homogenous nation with exceptions: Prejudice and its ideology in Japanese society. In O. Feldman (Ed.) *Political psychology in Japan: Behind the nails that sometimes stick out (and get hammered down)* (pp.233-256). New York: Nova Science Publishers, Inc.

Mackie, V. (1998). Japayuki cinderella girl: Containing the immigrant other. *Japanese Studies, 18*(1), 45-63.

Mackie, V. (2010). Managing borders and managing bodies in contemporary Japan. *Journal of the Asia Pacific Economy, 15*(1), 71-85.

Makabe, T. (1979). Ethnic identity scale and social mobility: The case of Nisei in Toronto. *Canadian Review of Sociology and Anthropology, 16,* 136-145.

Marcia, J. (1966). Development and validation of ego-identity status. *Journal of Personality and Social Psychology, 3,* 551-558.

Marcia, J. (1980). Identity in adolescence. In J. Anderson (Ed.) *Handbook of adolescent psychology* (pp.159-187). New York: Wiley.

Marcia, J. (2010). Life transitions and stress in the context of psychosocial development. In T.W. Miller (Ed.) *Handbook of stressful transitions across the lifespan* (pp.19-34). New York: Springer.

McNeill, D. et al. (2009). Lowering the drawbridge on fortress Japan: Citizenship, nationality, and the rights of children. *Japan Focus, May 2009.* Retrieved June 22, 2009 from http://www.japanfocus.org/-Alex-Martin/3143

Moon, J.-S., & Mikami, H. (2009). Chiiki zaijyu nihonjin koreisha to zainichi korian koreisha no nento yoin no hikaku [Comparison of factors of falls between ethnic

Korean and Japanese older residents in an urban community in Japan]. *Nihon Ronen Igakkai Zasshi [Japanese Journal of Geriatrics], 46*(3), 232-238.

Moriizumi, S. (2011). Exploring identity negotiations: An analysis of intercultural Japanese-U.S. American families living in the United States. *Journal of Family Communication, 11*, 85-104.

Nakayama, M., & Hoshino, K. (2010). Development of the Multigroup Ethnic Identity Measure-Revised Japanese version. Poster presented at the 74th Annual Convention of the Japanese Psychological Association (Osaka, Japan).

Ong, A.D., Fuller-Rowell T.E., & Phinney, J.S. (2010). Measurement of ethnic identity: Recurrent and emergent issues. *Identity: An International Journal of Theory and Research, 10*, 39-49.

Phinney, J.S. (1990). Ethnic identity in adolescence and adulthood: A review of research. *Psychological Bulletin, 108*, 499-514.

Phinney, J.S. (1992). The Multigroup Ethnic Identity Measure: A new scale for use with diverse groups. *Journal of Adolescent Research, 7*(2), 156-176.

Phinney, J.S., & Ong, A.D. (2007). Conceptualization and measurement of ethnic identity: Current status and future directions, *Journal of Counseling Psychology, 54*, 271-281.

Piquero-Ballescas, M.-R. (2009). Global householding and care networks: Filipino women in Japan. *Asian and Pacific Migration Journal, 18*(1), 77-99.

Ponterotto, J.G., & Mallinckrodt, B. (2007). Introduction to the special section on racial and ethnic identity in counseling psychology: Conceptual and methodological challenges and proposed solutions. *Journal of Counseling Psychology, 54*, 219-223.

Ponterotto, J.G., & Park-Taylor, J. (2007). Racial and ethnic identity theory, measurement, and research in counseling psychology. *Journal of Counseling Psychology, 54*, 282-294.

Roberts, R.E., Phinney, J.S., Masse, L.C., Chen, Y.R., Roberts, C.R., & Romeo, A. (1999). The structure of ethnic identity of young adolescents from diverse ethnocultural groups. *Journal of Early Adolescence, 19*, 301-322.

Rosenthal, D.A., & Hrynevich, C. (1985). Ethnicity and ethnic identity: A comparative study of Greek-, Italian-, and Anglo-Australian adolescents. *International Journal of Psychology, 20*, 723-742.

Sugioka, M. & Kodama, K. (2005). Tainichi nikkei burajirujin no yokuutsu shojo to bunkateki shozokukan oyobi sapoto nettowaku no kanren [A study on the relationships between depressive symptoms and a sense of belonging to culture and social support networks of Japanese-Brazilians in Japan]. *Japanese Journal of Community Psychology, 9* (1), 1–13.

Tajfel, H. (1981). *Human groups and social categories.* Cambridge: Cambridge University Press.

Tanibuchi, S. (2009). Tainichi nikkei burazirujin no gakko tekio, oyako kankei oyobi chiiki sanka ni kansuru komyunithi shinrigakuteki chosa: Doitsu chiiki no nihonjin oyako tono hikaku wo chusin ni [A research of school adaptation, parent-child relationship and community participation among Japanese Brazilian living in Japan: Comparative study with Japanese]. *Annual Research Report of Graduate School of Education at Hiroshima University Part 3, 58,* 183-192.

Uematsu, A. (2010). Ibunka kankyo ni okeru minzoku identity no yakuwari: Shudan identity to jiga identity no kankei [The role of ethnic identity in cross-cultural environment: Relationship between group identity and ego identity]. *Personality Kenkyu [Japanese Journal of Personality], 19*(1), 25-37.

Umana-Taylor, A.J., Yazedjian, A., & Bamaca-Gomez, M. (2004). Developing the Ethnic Identity Scale using Eriksonian and social identity perspectives. *Identity: An International Journal of Theory and Research, 4,* 9-38.

World Bank (2012). *The World Bank open data.* Retrieved August 12, 2012 from http://data.worldbank.org/indicator.

Yoon, E. (2011). Measuring ethnic identity in the Ethnic Identity Scale and the Multigroup Ethnic Identity Measure-Revised. *Cultural Diversity and Ethnic Minority Psychology, 17*(2), 144-155.

Chapter 5 Ethnic Identity, Intergenerational Support, and Psychosocial Development among Younger and Older Adults in Japan

Kazumi Hoshino

INTRODUCTION

Transitions to Population and Family Diversity

In a global cross-border movement, immigrants and minorities have been facing challenges of acculturation worldwide. In particular, Japan has been historically considered a homogeneous nation. The percentage of immigrants of the total population was 1.7% in 2009, which was the lowest among industrialized countries (OECD, 2010). As Hoshino (2012a) notes, immigrants in Japan, who mainly come from China, South Korea, and Brazil, have been experiencing problems of social integration, and thus societal support to immigrants should be examined at each level of national, regional and local governments, communities, and among health care professionals. To form an international perspective, the International Social Survey Programme (ISSP: 2003) and the European Social Survey (ESS: 2008) investigated shaping beliefs concerning the consequences of immigration for the economy and cultural life among 23 European countries (ISSP), six countries of North America, Asia, Oceania, and 16 European countries (ESS). In general, younger, well-educated, urban residents were more likely to believe that immigration positively affects economy and cultural lives of the host countries. However, only Japan indicated that even well-educated people hold negative beliefs about the influence of immigration. Although nationals among other countries perceived greater benefits from immigration and were accepting of a more open immigration policy, Japan indicated the opposite trend which many Japanese nationals did not believe in the benefits of immigration and have maintained a strict immigration policy (OECD, 2010). These findings suggest that immigrants may have barriers to communication with Japanese nationals, and that immigrants may face prejudice as well as discrimination at all educational levels. Immigrants living in Japan need support in their striving for ethnic identity, and physical and mental health in their ethnic communities as well as society wide (Hoshino, 2012a).

However, dramatic changes of demography, policy, and economy have gradually influenced intergenerational support exchanges in family and sociocultural contexts in East Asian countries for the recent few decades. International migration and demographic changes including decreasing younger populations and increasing older populations have been affecting population and family diversity. Specifically Japan is facing increasing pressures for immigration to help meet the economic needs of an aging population and low birth rate. The resulting changes in diversity of the population may be associated with ethnic identity, which refers to the part of identity formation process that defines who he/she ethnically is and how he/she ethnically relates to diverse populations. This is the first study to identify predictors of ethnic identity in consideration of intergenerational support and psychosocial development among both younger and older adults in Japan.

Ethnic Identity Predictors: Psychosocial Development and Ethnic Identity

Identity consists of a hierarchy of positive and negative components throughout lifespan development that are culturally related. Minorities face the challenge of integrating features of a dominant culture with their original cultures, which are socially suppressed, in order to build ethnic identity (Erikson, 1968, 1980). Marcia (1966, 1980) developed a typology of identity status by individual crisis (i.e., exploring meaningful alternatives) and commitment (i.e., personal investment in what the individual does). Identity status shifts may occur in young adulthood, adulthood, and late life (Marcia, 2010). Although the identity process holds continuity between old constructs and new ones, new constructs expand life experiences and encompass commitments (Marcia & Simon, 2003). Ethnic identity is thought to develop throughout one's lifespan (Ong, Fuller-Rowell, & Phinney, 2010), and its main components include Exploration and Commitment (Phinney & Ong, 2007). Yoon (2011) provided theoretical evidence of the Multigroup Ethnic Identity Measure-Revised (MEIM-R) and demonstrated associations between combinations of the MEIM-R subscales and a typology of identity status.

In Japan there are very few studies of ethnic identity, and of those, very few use appropriate psychological measures. Uematsu (2010) revealed that Exploration was significant and positively associated with identity, and that Affirmation, Belonging, and Commitment was significant and negatively associated with identity among Japanese students living in the United States. In turn, identity was significant and positively associated with English language proficiency, adjustment to university life, familiarity with the host country, and students' physical and mental health. This finding suggests that ethnic identity exploration relates to identity among Japanese students as a minority in the United States. However, ethnic identity among native-born nationals has not been examined in Japan.

Although ethnic identity studies in the United States confirm a relation between ethnic identity and identity (Phinney, 1992; Roberts et al, 1999; Phinney & Ong, 2007), they have not focused on older populations and have not examined associations between ethnic identity and psychosocial development in late life. The present study viewed ethnic identity development as occurring throughout life and examined how psychosocial development of identity, integrity, generativity, and gerotranscendence affected ethnic identity. Generativity comprises comprehensive attitudes towards procreativity, creativity, and productivity (Erikson & Erikson, 1997), bridges generations of diverse ethnic groups, and fosters ethnic knowledge and cultural values. Thus, the author takes into consideration that generativity may promote development of ethnic identity as well as overall identity. Integrity relates to an individual reflection on his/her life, including how he/she integrates life with death in a way that reflects ethnically defined basic attitudes towards end of life issues. Integrity may relate to ethnic identity in this regard.

In terms of psychosocial development in later life, Erikson & Erikson (1997) discussed transcendence as a potential ninth stage of psychosocial development. Transcendence is hypothesized to allow people to confront dystonic states and fear of death as independent of the universe and time. Tornstam (1996a, 1996b, 2005) defined gerotranscendence as a psychosocial development among the oldest old population (85 years and older) and proposed a category structure from interview data. The Cosmic Dimension held subcategories such as connections to earlier generations, and life and death. The Dimension of the Self contained body-transcendence, self-transcendence, and ego-integrity. The Dimension of Social and Personal Relationships held changed meaning and importance of relations, and everyday wisdom. These dimensions each correspond to the Cosmic, Coherence, and Solitude Dimensions of the Gerotranscendence Scale Type 2 (Tornstam, 1997a, 1997b, 2005). Life satisfaction and social support each have significant and positive associations to the Cosmic, and the Coherence Dimensions among older adults in Sweden (Tornstam, 2005). Thus, gerotranscendence functions as ego integrity beyond fear of death, and body and self transcendence, and therefore may be associated with ethnic identity in the context of historical succession of human beings.

Intergenerational Support and Ethnic Identity

Historically Japanese nationals have emphasized familialism norms based on Confucianist and Buddhist beliefs, which are similar to norms in other East Asian countries. However, a shift from family care to institutional care has accelerated since Long-Term Care Insurance was introduced in 2000. Also, women are more likely to develop voluntary relationships with their biological mothers than with their mothers-in-law, while some older adults in their eighties and nineties, particularly in rural regions, expect caregiving from their children and grandchildren (Arai, Zarit, Sugiura, &Washio, 2002; Arai, 2000; Arai & Ikegami, 1998). In addition, as Kim, Zarit, & Han (2011) reported, rapid social and economic changes have affected such familialism norms and the structure of family intergenerational support exchanges between middle-aged adults and their parents/parents-in-law in South Korea. Only a minority of middle aged couples had traditional patterns of support, which emphasized the

114   Part 2   International Migration and Wellness Innovation in Japan

relationship with husband's parents. In addition, couples with non-traditional exchange patterns with parents had higher quality of marital relationships than did couples whose exchanges with parents derived from obligatory norms.

In the United States and European countries, researchers have investigated how ethnic socialization derives from learning about one's ethnic history, traditions, and cultural values from parents, grandparents, ancestors, and societies (Fingerman, Miller, Birditt, & Zarit, 2009; Fingerman, VanderDrift, Dotterer, Birditt, & Zarit, 2011; Birditt, Tighe, Fingerman, & Zarit, 2012; Gans, & Silverstein, 2006; Silverstein, Gans, Lowenstein, Giarruso, & Bengtson, 2010). Phinney, Ong, & Tanya (2000) demonstrated that cultural values of intergenerational family relationships was endorsed by middle-aged parents more than by adolescents among Armenians, Mexicans, and Vietnamese, and that discrepancies of the intergenerational values increased with the duration in the United States since migration. Although there are few studies that explore predictors of ethnic identity in family and community contexts, Juang & Nguyen (2010) identified predictors of ethnic identity among Chinese American college students. Parents' family obligation beliefs were significant and positively associated with Ethnic Engagement (i.e., exploration and behavioral engagement with one's ethnic group), and Ethnic Pride (i.e., positive feelings towards one's ethnic groups). Cultural Resources (i.e., cultural support from one's ethnic group) were significant and positively associated with Ethnic Engagement and Ethnic Clarity (i.e., a clear sense of and commitment to one's ethnic identity). Perceived discrimination was significant and positively related to Ethnic Engagement but negatively to Ethnic Pride. This outcome showed that family obligation beliefs, community resources, and perceived

Chapter 5 Ethnic Identity, Intergenerational Support, and Psychosocial Development among Younger and Older Adults in Japan   115

hardships were significant predictors of ethnic identity. However, associations between intergenerational support exchanges, psychosocial development, and ethnic identity have not been clarified.

These findings suggest that researchers should deepen their understanding of interactions between ethnic identity, intergenerational support, and social contexts in light of rapid changes in demography, economics, and social policies. Much of the research with ethnic identity has focused on immigrants, but less is known about the processes in native-born persons and older adults. In the studies above, ethnic differences and cultural values were regarded as independent variables, and intergenerational support was regarded as a dependent variable. Since there are seldom studies on ethnic identity in Japan, not to mention those which also focus on older adults, researchers should first explore predictors of ethnic identity among native-born nationals.

Physical and Functional Factors

Since the present study focuses on older adults, the author considers physical and functional predictors as potential contributors to ethnic identity based on the Disablement Process Model. Nagi (1979, 1991) developed the original model, and Verbrugge and Jette (1994) proposed the Disablement Process Model. This model explains how a main path way, including pathology (i.e., disease and injury), functional impairments (i.e., dysfunctions in specific body systems), and functional limitations (i.e., restrictions in basic physical and mental actions), may relate to future disability. The model also describes how risk factors (i.e., predisposing characteristics), extraindividual factors (i.e., physical, and social environments), and intraindividual factors (i.e., changes in lifestyles and behaviors) may affect a main path way and future disability.

Based on the model, previous studies have clarified variables that were associated with disability in very late life: Disease level as pathology; Vision, grip strength, and lung functioning as functional impairments; Physical limitations, cognition and memory, and pain as functional limitations; ADL and IADL as disability; and Subjective health, social support, depression, and mastery as intraindividual factors (Femia, Zarit, & Malmberg, 2001; Fauth, Zarit, Malmberg, & Johansson, 2007; Zarit, Griffiths, & Berg, 2004). The strength of the model is to incorporate social, psychological, and environmental contexts into physical, and functional variables for a comprehensive understanding of individual differences in disability.

This study examined associations between physical factors, and functional factors, and ethnic identity. Physical traits and appearance have affected ethnic identity among different racial groups, in particular youth (Erikson, 1968, 1980; Phinney, 1992; Roberts et al., 1999), and functional variables have shaped group identity among diverse cultural groups, including people with disabilities (Banks, 2006). With the author's best knowledge, this research is the first study to shed light on ethnic identity among older adults and considers that aging may have influenced on ethnic identity. According to physical and functional declines, older adults may have opportunities to review ethnic identity how these variables have changed how they have lived as one of ethnic groups and to reorganize ethnic identity as a membership of one's ethnic group.

Present Study

In summary, there are few intergenerational comparative studies of ethnic identity. Also, research that clarifies associations between ethnic identity

Chapter 5 Ethnic Identity, Intergenerational Support, and Psychosocial Development among Younger and Older Adults in Japan   117

and intergenerational relationships, in particular intergenerational support exchanges between younger and older adults, may be particularly important, in light of current demographic changes toward increasing diversity. In addition, associations between ethnic identity and psychosocial development, specifically from adulthood through later life, should be identified, since previous studies addressed only relationships between ethnic identity and identity in adolescence. The goal of this study was to explore the association of intergenerational support exchanges and psychosocial development of identity, generativity, integrity, and gerotranscendence with ethnic identity among younger and older adults in Japan, by adding physical and functional factors.

In addition, as the present study targeted active community-dwelling older adults, the author emphasized relationships between functional limitations and future disability which were influenced by risk factors and intraindividual factors. In consideration of the Disablement Process Model and previous studies, this study selected independent variables to explore predictors of ethnic identity: Limitations due to health mobility and pain as functional limitations; ADL and IADL as future disability; Subjective health, intergenerational support, depression, and psychosocial development as intraindividual factors; and Participants' social characteristics as risk factors.

METHODS

Participants

Four hundred forty three Japanese participants included 203 younger adults (114 men, 89 women) and 240 community-dwelling older adults (130

118   Part 2   International Migration and Wellness Innovation in Japan

men, 110 women). The mean age of younger adults was 19.28 years old (SD=1.04), and that of older adults was 69.25 years old (SD=4.78). At one University, 235 students agreed to participate in a questionnaire of an international research project in their classes, if they agreed. At the Senior Citizen College, 525 older adults answered a questionnaire during their classes upon their agreement, and 271 older adults returned questionnaires by mail. The questionnaires of 32 younger adults and 31 older adults were removed from data because they contained more than one-third missing items on each one scale that we mentioned below. The respondent rate was 86.38% among younger adults, 45.71% among older adults, and 58.29% among the total participants, respectively. The Senior Citizen College was a lifelong learning institute in central Japan in which older adults lived independently in their communities and could attend at least two days of courses per week.

The present study was approved by the Institutional Review Board of the Senior Citizen College. If the participants agreed to participate in a questionnaire of an international research project, they signed the informed consent. The project members kept questionnaires confidential and excluded individual indentifying information from data by coding with participants' IDs.

Measures

Dependent Variables: Ethnic Identity: To measure ethnic identity, this study selected the Multigroup Ethnic Identity Measure-Revised (MEIM-R: Phinney & Ong, 2007), which was developed from the original MEIM (Phinney, 1992). The MEIM-R had a two-factor structure: Exploration (three items); and Commitment (three items). For development of the

Chapter 5 Ethnic Identity, Intergenerational Support, and Psychosocial Development among Younger and Older Adults in Japan   119

Japanese version (Nakayama & Hoshino, 2010), a bilingual researcher of psychology translated the MEIM and MEIM-R from English into Japanese, and another bilingual researcher independently made the back-translation. Next, the two researchers discussed translation accuracy of the MEIM and MEIM-R. Finally, Professors Jean S. Phinney and Anthony D. Ong gave the author permission to use the translated versions as Japanese versions of the MEIM and MEIM-R. The Japanese version rated items in the same way as the original, using a five-point scale from 1 (strongly disagree) to 5 (strongly agree). A similar two-factor structure was found: Exploration; and Commitment, though with one difference, that item 3 "I understand pretty well what my ethnic group membership means to me" loaded on Exploration, not Commitment. The scales had good internal reliability (Cronbach's alpha) and validity was confirmed due to the correspondence between the subscales and identity status (Marcia, 1980).

Independent Variables: Psychological Factors: Psychosocial Development, and Depression: In consideration of the Disablement Process Model, this study selected independent variables and their measures to assess intraindividual factors (i.e., physical, social, and psychological factors), functional limitations, future disability, and risk factors. In terms of psychological factors, the author chose the Erikson's Psychological Stage Inventory (EPSI) to measure identity, generativity, and integrity. The EPSI (Rosenthal, Gurney, & Moore, 1981) evaluates psychosocial development from infancy to young adulthood, and the Japanese Version (Nakanishi, Mizuno, Furuichi, & Sakata, 1985; Nakanishi & Sakata, 2001) was developed to assess psychosocial development from adulthood to later life. Of the 56 items, the author used only Identity (six

120   Part 2   International Migration and Wellness Innovation in Japan

items), Generativity (six items), and Integrity (seven items), which were most relevant to an adult population. Items were rated on a five-point scale from 1 (strongly disagree) to 5 (strongly agree).

The author used the Gerotranscendence Scale Type 2 (GST2: 10 items: Tornstam, 1997a, 1997b, 2005) to evaluate gerotranscendence as psychosocial development in very late life. The Japanese version (Hoshino, Zarit, & Nakayama, 2012) had a three-factor structure, including the Cosmic, the Coherence, and the Solitude Dimensions, with omission of item 1 that was originally reported by Tornstam, rated on a four-point scale from 1 (disagree) to 4 (agree).

The Japanese version of the CES-D (Radloff, 1977; Shima, Shikano, Kitamura, & Asai, 1985; Shima, 1998) was used to measure depression. In the original version, 20 items were rated on a four-point scale: 1 (rarely or none of the time, i.e. < 1 day); 2 (some of the time, i.e. 1-2 days); 3 (occasionally, i.e. 3-4 days); and 4 (most of the time, i.e. 5-7 days).

Independent Variables: Social Factor: Intergenerational Social Support: To assess intergenerational support, the author selected the Intergenerational Support Scale (ISS: Fingerman et al., 2009). The ISS estimated intergenerational support exchanges between adult parents and their grown children, rated on a seven-point scale. The Japanese version (Hoshino & Zarit, 2013) was modified to evaluate support exchanges between younger generations and older adults. Of the 13 items in the ISS for young adults, receiving support from the older person to whom they felt closest (six items), rated on a three-point scale: 1 (never); 2 (sometimes); and 3 (always); providing support (six items), rated on a three-point scale: 1 (never); 2 (sometimes); and 3 (always); and health status of the older person

Chapter 5   Ethnic Identity, Intergenerational Support, and Psychosocial Development among Younger and Older Adults in Japan   121

to whom they felt closest (one item), rated on a five-point scale from 1 (poor) to 5 (excellent). The ISS for older adults also included the 13 items and asked them about the younger person to whom they felt closest. In addition, the participants rated the relationship's importance (one item) on a five-point scale: 1 (most important older person or younger person in your life); 2 (among the three most important; 3 (among the 10 most important); 4 (among the 20 most important); and 5 (less important than that), respectively.

Independent Variables: Physical Factor: Subjective Health: A physical factor centered on subjective health, and the author used two items from the Short-Form-36 Health Survey Version 2 (SF-36, Version 2: Medical Outcomes Trust, Health Assessment Lab, & Quality Metric Inc., 2002; Quality Metric Inc., & Fukuhara, 2002), rated on a five-point scale from 1 (excellent) to 5 (poor).

Independent Variables: Functional Limitations: Limitations due to Health Mobility and Pain: To measure functional limitations, this study highlighted limitations due to health mobility and pain perception. The author used five items of limitations due to health mobility from the SF-36 Version 2, rated on a two-point scale: 1 (yes); and 2 (no). Two items of pain from the SF-36 Version 2 were rated on a six-point scale from 1 (none) to 6 (very severe).

Independent Variables: Future Disability: ADL and IADL: The present study focused on ADL and IADL as future disability. To measure ADL, five items of ADL were used from the SF-36 Version 2 , rated on a three-point

122   Part 2   International Migration and Wellness Innovation in Japan

scale; 1 (yes, limited a lot); 2 (yes, limited a little); and 3 (no, not limited at all). This study selected the IADL Section of the OARS Multidimensional Functional Assessment Questionnaire: Fillenbaum, 1998) to evaluate IADL and developed the Japanese version (Hoshino & Zarit, 2013). The author used seven items, rated on a three-point scale: 0 (without help); 2 (with some help); and 3 (dependent).

Risk Factors: Social Characteristics: Risk factors referred to participants' social characteristics, and were rated as follows. Marital status on a scale ranging from 1 (married), 2 (never-married), 3 (widowed), and 4 (divorced); current job status on a scale ranging from 1 (unemployed), 2 (full-time job), and 3 (part-time job); living arrangement on a scale ranging from 1 (living alone), and 2 (living with families/others); housing on a scale ranging 1 (their own home), and 2 (support apartment). They also answered age, gender, the numbers of their children and of grandchildren, years of education and of their past job careers. The author coded gender as 1 (women), 0 (men); marital status as 1 (married), 0 (not married); current job status 1 (full-time/part-time jobs), 0 (unemployment); living arrangement as 1 (living with families/others), 0 (living alone); housing as 1 (living in support apartment), 0 (living in their home); and age, each year of education and past job careers, and the number of children and of grandchildren.

Data Analysis

The author calculated Pearson's correlations between the MEIM-R, other scales, and participants' social characteristics. A multiple regression analysis with simultaneous entry of variables was performed to identify predictors of ethnic identity. The present study used the SPSS Version 18.

RESULTS

Participants' Social Characteristics

As can been seen in Table 5-1, 2.0 % of younger adults and 77.9 % of older adults were married. The mean of years of their education and their past job careers were 12.73 years (SD=1.68) and 0.9 years (SD=0.78) among younger adults, and 13.23 years (SD=2.69) and 31.71 years (SD=16.71) among older adults, respectively. Unemployment rate was 58.6% among younger adults. Among older adults, 85.5% were not employed, mainly due to retirement. With regard to living arrangement, 60.1% of younger adults and 12.9% of older adults lived alone.

Correlations Between the MEIM-R And Other Variables

Calculating Pearson's correlations for all variables (Table 5-2), the author selected independent variables for the multiple regression analysis by deleting variables with no significant correlations to Exploration or Commitment of the MEIM-R among both groups. Excluded variables were relationship importance, and health status of the most familiar younger/older person of the ISS, instrumental activities of daily living of the OARS Multidimensional Functional Assessment Questionnaire, activities of daily living, subjective health, pain, limitations due to health mobility of the SF-36 Version 2, and participants' social characteristics except age and gender. Consequently, independent variables consisted of Identity, Generativity, and Integrity of the EPSI, the Cosmic, the Coherence, and the Solitude Dimensions of the GST2, the CES-D, receiving and providing intergenerational support of the ISS, age, and gender. Dependent variables included Exploration and Commitment.

124   Part 2   International Migration and Wellness Innovation in Japan

Table 5-1 The Participants' Social Characteristics

Social Characteristics	Younger Adults (N=203)	Older Adults (N=240)
Age, M (SD)	19.28 (1.04)	69.25 (4.78)
Gender, Proportion (%)		
Men	114 (56.2%)	130 (54.2%)
Women	89 (43.8%)	110 (45.8%)
Marital Status, Proportion (%)		
Married	4 (2.0%)	187 (77.9%)
Never Married	199 (98.0%)	3 (1.3%)
Widowed	0 (0%)	37 (15.4%)
Divorced	0 (0%)	13 (5.4%)
Children, Proportion (%)		
Yes	0 (0%)	226 (94.2%)
No	203 (100%)	14 (5.8%)
The Number of Children, M (SD)	0 (0)	2.09 (0.86)
Grandchildren, Proportion (%)		
Yes	0 (0%)	182 (75.8%)
No	203 (100%)	58 (24.2%)
The Number of Grandchildren, M (SD)	0 (0)	2.26 (1.82)
Years of Education, M (SD)	12.73 (1.68)	13.23 (2.69)
Years of Job Careers, M (SD)	0.09 (0.78)	31.71 (16.71)
Current Job, Proportion (%)		
Unemployed	119 (58.6%)	206 (85.8%)
Full Time Job	2 (1.0%)	9 (3.8%)
Part Time Job	73 (36.0%)	25 (10.4%)
No answer	9 (4.4%)	0 (0%)
Living Arrangement, Proportion (%)		
Living Alone	122 (60.1%)	31 (12.9%)
Living with Families/Others	77 (37.9%)	208 (86.7%)
No answer	4 (2.0%)	1 (0.4%)
Housing, Proportion (%)		
Living in Their Own Home	158 (77.8%)	237 (98.8%)
Support Apartment	2 (1.0%)	3 (1.3%)
No answer	43 (21.2%)	0 (0%)

Chapter 5　Ethnic Identity, Intergenerational Support, and Psychosocial Development among Younger and Older Adults in Japan　125

Table 5-2 Correlations between the MEIM-R and Other Variables

	Exploration	Commitment	Exploration	Commitment
	Younger Adults	(N=203)	Older Adults	(N=240)
Cosmic Dimension	.40***	.23***	.39***	.26***
Coherence Dimension	.09	.04	.19**	.14*
Solitude Dimension	-.12*	-.04	-.21***	-.19***
Identity	.13*	.07	.33***	.30***
Generativity	.30***	.12*	.39***	.30***
Integrity	-.03	.03	.22***	.25***
Providing Support	-.16*	-.11	-.15**	.01
Receiving Support	.11	.01	.14*	.24***
The CES-D	-.06	-.09	-.14*	-.11*
Age	.09	.06	.18**	.19***
Gender a	.07	.02	-.08	-.03

Note: The MEIM-R=The Multigroup Ethnic Identity Measure-Revised; The GST2=The Gerotranscendence Scale Type 2; The EPSI=The Erikson's Psychological Stage Inventory; The ISS=The Intergenerational Support Scale; The CES-D=The Center for the Epidemiologic Studies Depression Scale.

a　gender (0=men; 1=women).

* $p < .05$; ** $p < .01$; *** $p < .001$.

Table 5-3 Multiple Regression Analysis of Ethnic Identity of Younger Adults and Older Adults

Independent Variables	Dependent Variables (B) The MEIM-R	
	Exploration	Commitment
Younger Adults		
Cosmic Dimension	.34***	.21**
Generativity		.25**
Integrity	-.17*	
R^2	.20***	.02
Older Adults		
Cosmic Dimension	.31***	.18***
Identity	.20*	.20*
Generativity	.26**	.16*
Receiving support		.18**
R^2	.27***	

Note: Dependent variables; The subscales of the Multigroup Ethnic Identity Measure-Revised.

Independent variables; The GST2=The Gerotranscendence Scale Type 2; The EPSI =The Erikson's Psychological Stage Inventory; The ISS=The Intergenerational Support Scale; The CES-D=The Center for the Epidemiologic Studies Depression Scale; and Social Characteristics (age, gender).

* $p < .05$; ** $p < .01$; *** $p < .001$.

Chapter 5 Ethnic Identity, Intergenerational Support, and Psychosocial Development among Younger and Older Adults in Japan   127

Multiple Regression Analysis

A multiple regression analysis with simultaneous entry of variables was performed to explore association of intergenerational support exchanges and psychosocial development with ethnic identity for each group of younger and older adults in Japan (Table 5-3). Among younger adults, the Cosmic Dimension ($B=.34$, $p < .001$) and Generativity ($B=.25$, $p < .01$) were significant and positively associated with Exploration, while Integrity ($B= -.17$, $p < .05$) was significant and negatively associated with it. The Cosmic Dimension ($B=.21$, $p < .01$) was significant and positively associated with Commitment. Among older adults, the Cosmic Dimension ($B=.31$, $p < .001$), Identity ($B=.20$, $p < .05$), and Generativity ($B=.26$, $p < .01$) were significant and positively associated with Exploration. The Cosmic Dimension ($B=.18$, $p < .01$), Identity ($B=.20$, $p < .05$), and receiving intergenerational support ($B=.16$, $p < .05$) were significant and positively associated with Commitment.

DISCUSSION

This study showed that indicators of psychosocial development were associated with ethnic identity in both younger and older adults. Identity had significant and positive associations with Exploration and Commitment of ethnic identity among older adults. This implies that older adults have established identity, and that identity contributed to exploring undeveloped aspects of ethnic identity and furthered commitment to one's ethnic group. However, identity did not show associations with any aspect of ethnic identity among younger adults. In contrast, American studies reported relations between ethnic identity, identity status (Yoon, 2011), and self-esteem among youth (Phinney, 1992; Roberts et al., 1999). Taking these studies into consideration, these results reflect that Japanese people emphasize harmony with others over establishing their own unique identity (Hoshino, 2001). According to an international comparative study, Japanese nationals tend to highlight their identity less clearly than Americans and Swedes (Hoshino, 2012b). This characteristic may be found particularly among younger adults (Marcus & Kitayama, 1991, 2003), for whom peer group relationships are paramount. They prioritize others in their homogenous communities and suppress development of identity as well as ethnic identity.

Generativity (i.e., procreativity, creativity and productivity) was significant and positively associated with Exploration among younger adults and older adults. Traditionally, Japan has been considered as having a tendency to respect older generations and emphasize intergenerational ties between their ancestors and descendants (Hoshino, 2001, 2012b; Araki, 2011). Hoshino, Zarit, & Nakayama (2013) clarified that Japanese youth were concerned about caring for older generations and expected to be taken care by future generations. Reflecting these interactive intergenerational relationships, ethnic values and practices are maintained between younger and older generations, and therefore generativity may enhance exploration of an individual ethnic life among older adults as well as younger adults in Japan.

Of gerotranscendence, only the Cosmic Dimension (i.e., connections to earlier generations, and life and death) had significant and positive associations with Exploration and Commitment among younger and older adults. Perceived relationships with earlier generations at a meta-level may strengthen not only Exploration of how an individual behaves ethnically but also Commitment to an ethnic investment in the historical, social, and cultural backgrounds among both groups. As Yamada and Kato (2006) suggested, Japanese younger adults had stronger concerns of a generative lifecycle image, life, and death than German, French, and Vietnamese. Taku, Calhoun, Tedeschi, Gil-Rivas, Kilmer, and Cann (2007) also pointed out that Japanese college students had an interest in spirituality and appreciated to be supported by diverse generations. This sample may also be familiar with a sense of connection to earlier generations and opportunities to think about life and death, and it had significant and positive associations with Exploration and Commitment of ethnic identity.

However, the Coherence Dimension (i.e., body-transcendence, self-transcendence, and ego-integrity) did not show any significant associations with Exploration and Commitment among either group. This sample of older adults may be in the middle of such developmental tasks of reintegrating their identity. Similarly, younger adults are in the process of developing identity, and they may not have developed sufficiently for the Coherence Dimension. The Solitude Dimension (i.e., changed meaning of important relationships, and everyday wisdom) also did not have associations with any aspect of ethnic identity among either group. It is considered that the definition includes different developmental constructs, and so the Solitude Dimension may not show direct associations with ethnic identity.

In terms of intergenerational support, only receiving support from younger generations was significant and positively associated with Commitment among older adults. As Juang & Nguyen (2010) reported, cultural resources (i.e., support from one's ethnic group) were associated with Ethnic Clarity (i.e., ethnic commitment) among Chinese American youth. This study demonstrated that among older adults, receiving support from younger generations may promote commitment to ethnic identity as older adults reflect on their lives and how they ethnically relate to others. However, among younger adults, receiving support was not significantly associated with any aspect of ethnic identity. They are considered to be in the process of identity formation and have less opportunity to struggle with ethnic identity when they communicate with older adults. Also, providing support, whether to younger or older adults, was not significantly associated with ethnic identity among either group. This outcome indicates that, in general, exploration of ethnic identity does not necessarily require providing intergenerational support among younger and older adults at their daily life level as a majority in Japan.

On the other hand, this study did not reveal significant correlations between functional limitations (limitations due to health mobility and pain), future disability (ADL and IADL), a physical factor (subjective health), and the two factors of ethnic identity in Pearson's correlations. Since previous studies on ethnic identity (Phinney, 1992; Roberts et al., 1999; Juang & Nguyen, 2010; Yoon, 2011) have not targeted older adults, these studies have not dealt with physical and functional factors. In this study, the participants were healthy community-dwelling older adults who may not have had opportunities to meditate on how they ethnically live in the face of serious diseases and functional decline. Also, among the healthier Swedish oldest old population, social network, self-rated health, sense of control, and depression were significantly related to life satisfaction however physical health and cognitive functioning were not (Berg, Hassing, McClearn, & Johansson, 2006). This healthier sample had more years of education and higher past job status than a large sample might have had (Yong and Saito,

2012). These differences in the sample may have contributed to our findings that neither functional nor physical factors had any significant correlations to Exploration and Commitment of ethnic identity.

Limitations and Future Directions

The present study holds several limitations. First, the sample is not nationally representative, nor are grandchildren and grandparents drawn from the same families. Older generations consisted of students at the Senior Citizen College, and younger adults included only university students. Second, the response rate of younger adults was higher than that of older adults. Although younger adults received and answered the questionnaires in their classes, older adults received them in their classes and returned the questionnaires by mail. Such a difference in the method may have affected the low response rate among older adults. Third, ethnic identity formation throughout lifespan development may be clarified including childhood and young adulthood with a longitudinal research design. Finally, researchers should compare ethnic identity between Japanese nationals and immigrants in Japan, as minorities are assumed to have specific ethnic identity formation because of exclusion and discrimination. Future research needs to determine interactions between ethnic identity and intergenerational support exchanges by using a population-based sample composed of adolescents, adults, and elderly parents of both nationals and immigrants.

CONCLUSION

This study explored the association of intergenerational support exchanges

132   Part 2   International Migration and Wellness Innovation in Japan

and psychosocial development of identity, generativity, integrity, and gerotranscendence with ethnic identity among younger and older adults in Japan. Among younger adults, the Cosmic Dimension and Generativity each had significant positive associations with Exploration, and the Cosmic Dimension had a significant positive association with Commitment. Among older adults, the Cosmic Dimension, Identity, and Generativity each had significant and positive associations with Exploration. The Cosmic Dimension, Identity, and receiving intergenerational support each had significant and positive associations with Commitment. Thus, the present study demonstrates interesting predictors of ethnic identity among younger and older adults in Japan. Future research needs to examine ethnic identity development from adolescence to later life by using a population-based data of youth, adult, and older generations, given unprecedented international demographic and social changes.

ACKNOWLEDGMENTS

This study was partly presented at the 63 rd Annual Scientific Meeting of the Gerontological Society of America in New Orleans, LA (Hoshino, et al., 2010). The author wishes to thank Professors Jean S. Phinney and Anthony D. Ong for permitting the author to use the Japanese version of the MEIM-R. The author also appreciates Dr. Steven H. Zarit for his suggestions. In addition, the author acknowledges the participants at the Senior Citizen College and research assistants, including Mr. Makoto Nakayama and Ms. Hiromi Kitagawa. This study was funded by the Grant-In-Aid for Scientific Research of the Japan Society for the Promotion of Science (Principal Investigator: Kazumi Hoshino).

REFERENCES

Arai, Y. (2000). Challenges of an aging society in Japan. *Registered Home and Services*, 4, 182-184.

Arai, Y., & Ikegami, N. (1998). How will Japan cope with the impending surge of dementia? In A.W.B. Winblad, B. Jonsson, & G. Karlson (Eds.) *The health economics of dementia.* Chichester: Wiley.

Arai, Y., Zarit, S.H., Sugiura, M., & Washio, M. (2002). Patterns of outcome of caregiving for the impaired elderly: A longitudinal study in Japan. *Aging and Mental Health*, 6, 39-46.

Araki, M. (2011). Tokubetsu yogo rojin homu shokuin no jenerathibithi to shigoto no yunoukan no kanren [Relationship between care staff generativity and perceived job competence in elderly nursing homes], *Nihon Ronen Igakkaishi [Japanese Journal of Geriatrics]*, 48, 679-685.

Banks, J. A. (2006). *Cultural diversity and education: Foundations, curriculum, and teaching* (5th ed.). Boston: Pearson Education.

Berg, A.I., Hassing, L.B., McClearn, G.E., & Johansson, B. (2006). What matters for life satisfaction in the oldest old? *Aging and Mental Health*, 10, 275-264.

Birditt, K.S., Tighe, L.A., Fingerman, K.L., & Zarit, S.H. (2012). Intergenerational relationship quality across three generations, *The Journals of Gerontology: Psychological Sciences and Social Sciences*, 67, 627-638.

Erikson, E.H. (1968). *Identity and the life cycle.* New York: W. W. Norton & Company.

Erikson, E.H. (1980). *Identity: Youth and crisis.* New York: W. W. Norton & Company.

Erikson, E.H., & Erikson, J.M. (1997). *The life-cycle completed (extended version).* New York: W. W. Norton & Company.

European Social Survey (2008). The European Social Survey Programme 2002. Retrieved July 10, 2012 from http://dx.doi.org/10.1787/884783236554

Fauth, E.B., Zarit, S.H., Malmberg, B., & Johansson, B. (2007). Physical, cognitive, and psychological variables from the disablement process model predict patterns of independence and the transition into disability for the oldest-old, *The Gerontologist*, 47, 613-624.

Femia, E.E., Zarit, S.H., & Johansson, B. (2001). The disablement process in very late life: A study of the oldest-old in Sweden, *The Journals of Gerontology Series B: Psychological Sciences*, 56B, 12-23.

Fillenbaum, G. (1998). *Multidimensional functional assessment of older adults: The Duke Older Americans Resources and Services procedures.* Hillsdale, NJ: Lawrence Erlbaum Associates.

Fingerman, K.L., Miller, L.M., Birditt, K.S., & Zarit, S.H. (2009). Giving to the good and the needy: Parental support of grown children, *Journal of Marriage and Family*, 71, 1220-1233.

Fingerman, K.L., VanderDrift, L.E., Dotterer, A.M., Birditt, K.S., & Zarit, S.H. (2011). Support to aging parents and grown children in Black and White families, *The Gerontologist*, 51, 441-452.

Gans, D., & Silverstein, M. (2006). Norms of filial responsibility for aging parents across time and generations, *Journal of Marriage and Family*, 68, 961-976.

Hoshino, K. (2012a). Healthy aging among older immigrants in Japan. In A.E. Scharlach & K. Hoshino (Eds.) *Healthy aging in sociocultural context* (pp.72-81). New York: Routledge.

Hoshino, K. (2012b). Sociocultural support model for healthy aging for older immigrants: Perspectives from the United States, Sweden, and Japan. In A.E. Scharlach & K. Hoshino (Eds.) *Healthy aging in sociocultural context* (pp.85-96). New York: Routledge.

Hoshino, K., Zarit, S.H., & Nakayama, M. (2012). Development of the Gerotranscendence Scale Type 2: Japanese version, *International Journal of Aging and Human Development*, 75, 217-237.

Hoshino, K., Zarit, S.H., & Nakayama, M. (2013). Lifecycle images and psychosocial development among adolescents in Japan, *Central Japanese Journal of Psychology*, 7, 11-21.

International Social Survey Programme (2003). *The International Social Survey Programme 2003.* Retrieved July 10, 2012 from http://dx.doi.org/10.1787/884768681750

Juang, L.P., & Nguyen, H.H. (2010). Ethnic identity among Chinese-American youth: The role of family obligation and community factors on ethnic engagement, clarity, and pride, *Identity: An International Journal of Theory and Research*, 10, 20-38.

Kim, K., Zarit, S.H., & Han, G. (2011). The structure of intergenerational exchanges of middle-aged adults with their parents and parents-in-law in Korea. Poster presented at the 64 th Annual Scientific Meeting of the Gerontological Society of America (Boston, MA).

Marcia, J. (1966). Development and validation of ego-identity status, *Journal of Personality and Social Psychology,* 3, 551-558.

Marcia, J. (1980). Identity in adolescence. In J. Anderson (Ed.) *Handbook of adolescent psychology* (pp.159-187). New York: Wiley.

Marcia, J. (2010). Life transitions and stress in the context of psychosocial development. In T.W. Miller (Ed.) *Handbook of stressful transitions across the lifespan* (pp.19-34). New York: Springer.

Marcia, J., & Simon, F.U. (2003). Treading fearlessly: A commentary on personal persistence, identity development, and suicide, *Monographs of the Society for Research in Child Development,* 68, 131-181.

Marcus, H.R., & Kitayama, S. (1991). Culture and the self: Implications for cognition, emotion, and motivation, *Psychological Review,* 98, 224-253.

Marcus, H.R., & Kitayama, S. (2003). Culture, self, and the reality of the social, *Psychological Inquiry,* 14, 277-283.

Medical Outcomes Trust, Health Assessment Lab, & Quality Medical Inc. (2002). *SF-36 version 2.* Lincoln: The Medical Outcomes Trust, Health Assessment Lab, & Quality Medical Inc.

Nagi, S.Z. (1979). The concept and measurement of disability. In E.D. Berkowitz (Ed.) *Disability policies and government programs* (pp.1-15). New York: Praeger.

Nagi, S.Z. (1991). Disability concept revisited: Implications for prevention. In A.M. Pope & A.R. Tarlov (Eds.) *Disability in America: Toward a national agenda for prevention.* Washington, DC: National Academy Press.

Nakanishi, N., Mizuno, M., Furuichi, Y., & Sakata, T. (1985). *Identity no shinrigaku [Psychology of ego identity].* Tokyo: Yuhikaku.

Nakanishi, N., & Sakata, T. (2001) EPSI: Erikson shinri dankai mokuroku kensa [The EPSI: Erikson's Psychological Stage Inventory]. In I. Agari (Ed.) *Shinri assessment handbook dai ni han [Handbook of psychological assessment (2nd ed.)]* (pp. 365-367). Tokyo: Nishimura Shoten.

Nakayama, M., & Hoshino, K. (2010). Development of the Multigroup Ethnic Identity

Measure-Revised Japanese version. Poster presented at the 74 th Annual Convention of the Japanese Psychological Association (Osaka, Japan).

Organization of Economic Co-operation and Development (2010). *International migration outlook: The 2010 SOPEMI.* Paris: OECD.

Ong, A.D., Fuller-Rowell T.E., & Phinney, J.S. (2010). Measurement of ethnic identity: Recurrent and emergent issues, *Identity: An International Journal of Theory and Research,* 10, 39-49.

Phinney, J.S. (1992). The Multigroup Ethnic Identity Measure: A new scale for use with diverse groups, *Journal of Adolescent Research,* 7, 156-176.

Phinney, J.S., & Ong, A.D. (2007). Conceptualization and measurement of ethnic identity: Current status and future directions, *Journal of Counseling Psychology,* 54, 271-281.

Phinney, J.S., Ong, A.D., & Tanya, M. (2000). Cultural values and intergenerational value discrepancies in immigrant and non-immigrant families, *Child Development,* 71, 528-539.

Quality Medical Inc., & Fukuhara, S. (2002). *SF-36 Japanese version 2.* Tokyo: Quality Medical Inc.

Radloff, L.S. (1977). The CES-D scale: A self-report depression scale for research in the general population, *Applied Psychological Measurement,* 1, 385-401.

Roberts, R.E., Phinney, J.S., Masse, L.C., Chen, Y.R., Roberts, C.R., & Romeo, A. (1999). The structure of ethnic identity of young adolescents from diverse ethnocultural groups, *Journal of Early Adolescence,* 19, 301-322.

Rosenthal, D.A., Gurney, R.M., & Moore, S.M. (1981). From trust to intimacy: New inventory for examining Erikson's stage of psychosocial development, *Journal of Youth and Adolescence,* 510, 525-537.

Shima, S. (1998). *NIMH/CES-D Scale utsuby jiko hyoka shakudo [The CES-D Scale Japanese version: A self-report depression scale].* Tokyo: Chiba Test Center.

Shima, S., Shikano, T., Kitamura, T., & Asai, M. (1985). Atarashii yokuutsusei jiko hyoka shakudo ni tsuite [A new self-repot depression scale], *Psychiatry,* 27, 717-723.

Silverstein, M., Gans, D., Lowenstein, A., Giarruso, R., & Bengtson, V.L. (2010). Older parent-child relationships in six developed nations: Comparisons at the intersection of affection and conflict, *Journal of Marriage and Family,* 72, 1006-

1021.

Taku, K., Calhoun, L.G., Tedeschi, R.G., Gil-Rivas, V., & Kilmer, R.P., & Cann, A. (2007) Examining posttraumatic growth among Japanese university students, *Anxiety, Stress, & Coping*, 20, 353-367.

Tornstam, L. (1996a). Caring for the elderly: Introducing the theory of gerotranscendence as a supplementary frame of reference for caring for the elderly, *Scandinavian Journal of Caring Sciences*, 10, 144-150.

Tornstam, L. (1996b). Gerotranscendence: A theory about maturing into old age, *Journal of Aging and Identity*, 1, 37-50.

Tornstam, L. (1997a). Gerotranscendence: The contemplative dimension of aging, *Journal of Aging and Studies*, 11, 143-154.

Tornstam, L. (1997b). Gerotranscendence in a broad cross-sectional perspective, *Journal of Aging and Identity*, 2, 17-36.

Tornstam, L. (2005). *Gerotranscendence: A developmental theory of positive aging.* New York: Springer.

Uematsu, A. (2010). Ibunka kankyo ni okeru minzoku identity no yakuwari: Shudan identity to jiga identity no kankei [The role of ethnic identity in cross-cultural environment: Relationship between group identity and ego identity], *Japanese Journal of Personality*, 19, 25-37.

Verbrugge, L.M., & Jette, A.M. (1994). The disablement process, *Social Science and Medicine*, 38, 1-14.

Yamada, Y., & Kato, Y. (2006) Images of circular time and spiral repetition: The Generative Life Cycle Model, *Anxiety, Stress, & Coping*, 20, 353-367.

Yong, V., & Saito, Y. (2012). Are there education differentials in disability and mortality transitions and active life expectancy among Japanese older adults?: Findings from a 10 year prospective cohort study, *The Journals of Gerontology Series B: Psychological Sciences and Social Sciences*, 67B, 343-353.

Yoon, E. (2011). Measuring ethnic identity in the Ethnic Identity Scale and the Multigroup Ethnic Identity Measure-Revised. *Cultural Diversity and Ethnic Minority Psychology*, 17, 144-155.

Zarit, S.H., Griffiths, P.C., & Berg, S. (2004). Pain perceptions of the oldest old: A longitudinal study, *The Gerontologist*, 44, 459-468.

Part 3

Future Directions

Chapter 6 International Migration, Wellness, and Social Policies in the United States, Sweden, and Japan

Kazumi Hoshino

INTRODUCTION

Demographic Changes in International Aging Societies

This chapter will focus on healthy aging as wellness among older immigrants in the United States, Sweden, and Japan. The author will enlighten Asian immigrants, in particular Chinese immigrants who reflect global migration patterns. In 2014, the percentage of older adults of the total population was 14.0% in the United States, 20.0% in Sweden, 26.0% in Japan, and 9.0% in China (World Bank, 2015). However, because of rapid industrialization and economic development, there were huge differences within China. For example, the percentage of older adults of the total population was 14.1 % in Shanghai and 6.7% in Xinjiang in 2009 (National Bureau of Statistics of China, 2011). Also, in China the percentage is estimated to increase to 22.6% by 2040 (Kinsella & He, 2009).

Scharlach & Hoshino (2012) examined healthy aging in sociocultural contexts in the United States, Sweden, and Japan which are at the forefront of low fertility rates, declining labor forces, growing aging populations, and increasing migrants. As Hoshino (2012a) conducted international comparative research on healthy aging in the United States, Sweden, China, and Japan, the United States has been a diverse immigrant society and has

142   Part 3   Future Directions

been discussing a comprehensive federal health policy for elderly care. Sweden has been a homogeneous country, however the nation is gradually experiencing population diversity and has established a universal health care system. Japan has been an extremely homogeneous country and has been developing a national health policy and long-term care insurance. In China, with the controlled fertility rate due to the family planning policy of 1979, the family structure has been changing to one child-two parents-eight grandparents, and the Chinese government continues to legally define elderly care as the obligation of the older adults' children (Zhang, Guo, & Zheng, 2012). This perspective is based on Confucianism, incorporating parents' familism norms and children's filial piety. Structural health and income disparities has been expanded by a longstanding lack of national comprehensive social policy for elderly care, sufficient facilities for health and social services for older adults, and internal as well as external migration in rural regions, in particular (Lou & Gui, 2011). Although the Chinese government implemented health care reform in 2011, it is expected that remaining problems such as quality of care, education and training of medical professionals, and health insurance coverage need to be resolved (Eggleston, 2012). Under such circumstances, how will China as well as the United States, Sweden, and Japan provide care for the growing aging populations and older immigrants?

This chapter upholds three objectives. First, the author will analyze demographic changes and the most recent social policies for older adults and immigrants, including long-term care insurance in China (i.e., a migrant-sending country), and the United States, Sweden, and Japan (i.e., migrant-receiving countries). The author will also identify access and barriers to health care and social services among internal Chinese migrants

Chapter 6 International Migration, Wellness, and Social Policies in the United States, Sweden, and Japan   143

in China and international Chinese migrants in the United States, Sweden, and Japan. Second, the author will clarify associations between Chinese migration and healthy aging in China, the United States, Sweden, and Japan. Finally, the author will propose implications for social policies for elderly care among older Chinese immigrants in order to promote healthy aging in the context of global Chinese migration.

INTERNATIONAL CHINESE MIGRATION

Organisation for Economic Co-operation and Development (OECD, 2009) analyzed international migration and identified nine patterns of change: aging societies, talent shortages, demographic shifts, changing economic landscapes, political complexity, expanding business agendas, science-led innovation and growth, environmental risks, and global internet expansion. OECD (2009) also recommended that its members should consider the effects of global migration on key areas such as labor markets and local communities, including health care, schooling, and housing. Global cross-border geographic mobility reached its highest level in recorded history in 1995-2005. Naerssen, Spaan, & Zoomers (2008) suggested that global migration patterns were variously categorized, for example, permanent migrants, temporary migrants who are abroad on contract and stay for three to five years, and transient circular migrants who regularly return to their home. Chinese migration obviously reflects current international cross-border movement. Social policies in China as well as migrant receiving countries should promote healthy aging as an important global issue.

   Historically, out-migration from China has resulted from economic,

144   Part 3   Future Directions

political, and sociocultural factors (OECD, 2009). Rapid economic development for the past three decades has increased internal migration and has decreased the economic imperative for external migration. Future internal development, transparency, and democratization will affect economic and political factors. In the near future, Chinese migration to Japan and South Korea as well as to Russia will continue to increase. Also, migration is likely to continue to the United States, Canada, and the United Kingdom for academic purposes. In Sweden, the majority of migrants came from Iraq, Poland, Denmark, Finland, and China in 2010 (OECD, 2010). Globally Chinese have been migrating and immigrating to many countries, and manifesting the migration patterns mentioned earlier. These patterns continue to promote China's demographic, economic, and political powers to international societies, and settled Chinese migrants have been expanding their communities beyond China towns (Thuno, 2007). Returned migrants also have been bringing economic gains, higher job skills, and knowledge about different administrative systems to their original countries.

HEALTHY AGING

In terms of healthy aging, Rowe and Kahn (1987, 1988) defined the concept of successful aging as older adults who have "the ability to maintain three key behaviors or characteristics: low risk of disease and disease-related disability; high mental and physical function; and active engagement with life" (Rowe & Kahn, 1988, p.38). This concept has broadened to add other measures such as wisdom and resilience, to include older adults who adapt daily challenges in the face of ill health and declining functional abilities, and to expand understanding of physical environment and socioeconomic contexts. Therefore, the concept of healthy aging has emerged as a more suitable term than the original "successful aging," based on an ecological model (Satariano, 2006, 2012). Hoshino (2012b) proposed a Sociocultural Support Model of Healthy Aging for Older Immigrants by reflecting conceptual and empirical evidence from the United States, Sweden, and Japan. This model holds two directions: the Subjective Direction (subjective satisfaction); and the Objective Direction. It also has four dimensions: Physical, Social, Psychological, and Spiritual, and each dimension encompass both an objective and a subjective direction. The model emphasizes a subjective direction more than an objective one and considers healthy aging to be an ongoing process of adaptation that is a part of individual lifespan development, rather than an idealized goal. Strengths of this model are to transcend existing concepts of successful aging or healthy aging that focus on limited aspects of aging and are driven from deconceptualized perspectives (Scharlach & Hoshino, 2012).

SOCIAL POLICIES FOR ELDERLY CARE IN CHINA, THE UNITED STATES, SWEDEN, AND JAPAN

In this section, the author will examine Chinese internal and external migration and social policies for elderly care for the recent two decades in China (i.e., a migrant-sending country), as well as Chinese international migration and social policies in the United States, Sweden, and Japan, (i.e., migrant-receiving countries).

China

In terms of social policies for elderly care in China, the Protection of the

Rights and Interests of Older People was implemented in 1996 (Steering Committee of the National People's Congress of People's Republic of China, 1996; Lou & Gui, 2011). Although the Chinese government started a series of policies addressing the needs of the elderly (Liang, 1995; National News Office of People's Republic of China, 2006), the basic principle is a collaborative support system of four parties: the state, the community, the family, and the individual.

However, due to emerging long-term care needs along with an aging population, China has emphasized long-term care needs most recently in the guiding policy document, The Twelfth Five Year Plan for Aging Policy in Care System (China National Committee on Aging, 2011). This policy corresponds to the aging-in-place principle in which community resources and community services should be strengthened (Burgess & Burgess, 2006; China National Committee on Aging, 2011). As an example at the municipal level, the author sheds light on Shanghai's recent policy, the 2006 11 th Five Year Plan and the long-term care model (Shanghai Committee on Aging, 2006). In summary, challenges of social policies including huge regional differences in social policies for elderly care and health services among municipalities, particularly in rural regions, a lack of care facilities, and insufficient family caregiver support systems in China.

The United States

In the United States, the growing Hispanic, Latino, and Asian immigrants have accelerated demographic changes and population diversity (U.S. Census Bureau, 2011). The author will outline Medicare, which Congress enacted under Title XVIII of the Social Security Act in 1965 to provide tax-financed medical insurance for American older adults, as well as

Medicaid in which Congress enacted as an amendment to the existing Social Security Act in 1965 to provide health care to low-income people.

In 1965 Congress enacted Medicare under Title XVIII of the Social Security Act, providing tax-financed medical insurance for American older adults. In 1972 Congress expanded Medicare eligibility to younger people who have permanent disabilities and receive Social Security Disability Insurance (SSDI) and those who have end-stage renal disease (ESRD). In 2001Congress further expanded Medicare to cover younger people with ALS (Lou Gehrig's disease) (Barr, 2011).

Initially Medicare consisted exclusively of Part A, which covers hospital and other inpatient services, and Part B, which covers outpatient care, physician visits, and other medical services. Congress added Medicare Part C (Medicare Advantage), which allows enrollees to receive their benefits through a private plan under the Balanced Budget Act of 1997. Medicare Part D was created for prescription drugs under the Medicare Modernization Act of 2003.

All people 65 years and older who have been legal residents of the United States for at least five years are eligible for Medicare. People under 65 years old may also be eligible if they receive Social Security Disability Insurance (SSDI) benefits. Those who are 65 years and older must pay a monthly premium if they have not paid Medicare taxes over 10 years while working.

In 1965 Congress also enacted Medicaid, which provides health care to three groups who fall below the federal poverty line (FPL) and must be a U.S. citizen or legal immigrants depending on their entry dates; 1) members of low-income families with children; 2) elderly people who meet certain income requirements; and 3) disabled people. It is administered by the

148   Part 3   Future Directions

states, with the federal government reimbursing each state for a portion of program costs.

Many beneficiaries may qualify for Medicare and Medicaid. For a state Medicaid program to be eligible for reimbursement from the federal government, it must provide basic services to beneficiaries; 1) hospital care; 2) nursing home care; and 3) physician services, etc. States also have the options; 1) prescription drugs; and 2) home- and community-based care, etc.

In 2010 Patient Protection and Affordable Care Act (PPACA) was enacted. The aims of the Patient Protection and Affordable Care Act were to improve affordability of health insurance as well as lower uninsured percentage and to decrease health care costs of the government and individuals. The Patient Protection and Affordable Care Act may require reforming the private health insurance market and expanding the federal-state Medicaid program. However, people who work for small companies and undocumented residents remain uninsured.

Thus, historically a lack of federal elderly care policies may have expanded health disparities among older immigrants in which expensive health insurance systems lead to insufficient health care and growing the number of uninsured people. These inadequate policies and systems may cause shorter life expectancy by increasing incidence and prevalence of injury, chronic conditions, and diseases. The United States has underdeveloped a universal health care system among industrialized countries.

However, the Patient Protection and Affordable Care Act was enacted in 2010, and the uninsured percentage was decreased. On the other hand, immigrants and refugees, who do not fulfill the requirement, continue to face challenges to access to health care. Also, Medicare faces cost increases,

Chapter 6 International Migration, Wellness, and Social Policies in the United States, Sweden, and Japan   149

although Congress has made repeated efforts to constrain Medicare costs. Especially as the baby boomers become eligible for Medicare, the long-term financial viability is increasingly questioned (Barr, 2011).

Sweden

The main demographic trends in Sweden are the growing number of immigrant and elderly populations, in particular the oldest old populations (i.e., those 80 years and older). The Swedish universal health care and social welfare system has addressed that elderly care is a social right, and the elderly care has been regulated as an important local governmental task.

According to Edebalk (2010), in Sweden elderly care is a social right and has been regulated as important local governmental tasks. In 1992, a Community Care Reform was enacted, by which the municipalities were appointed the solo authority for all elderly care and home-based nursing. Also, the local authorities were paying the costs for elderly who were hospitalized but not in need of further medical treatment. Since then, the municipalities could no longer evade economic responsibility by requiring the county councils to cover costs. With these changes, the local governments were given more responsibility but also more freedom.

Currently, in the Swedish Social Services Act, the 290 municipalities decide elderly care. Financing of elderly care is mainly derived from the local taxes, and consumer fees are limited to a maximum level that finances 5% of the costs. Elderly care includes home help services and institutional or special-housing care, including old people's homes and nursing homes, etc.

Since 1990, municipalities reduced certain services and applied more strict needs-assessments. As a result, many older adults were purchasing

150   Part 3 Future Directions

market-based care services, and voluntary organizations were becoming involved in elderly care. In the last few years, local governments reduced institutional care and focused on home help services. 30 municipalities introduced a consumer-choice system. The user is free to choose a non-municipal care provider.

The demographic challenge of an aging population will affect the possibilities to finance elderly care. In particular, the oldest old populations, whose ages are 85 years and older, have been growing and will need more health services. Also, it is difficult for elderly caregivers to take care of their partners in their own homes (Socialstyrelsen, 2007). This may require Sweden to take financial responsibility for elderly care and introduce elderly care insurance.

Japan

The Japanese demographic changes in Japan includes a decreasing low fertility rate, a declining working age population, and an increasing elderly population, while the percentage of immigrants was the lowest among industrialized countries in 2010 (OECD, 2010). The author will summarize the Japanese national health care system and long-term insurance.

As Nakagawa & Gondo (2012) noted, in Japan the National Health Care Insurance Act' started in 1958 which provided comprehensive health care which most of people allowed to access medical services at low cost. The Act for the Welfare of the Aged of 1963 was enacted to include special nursing homes for frail older adults, and in 1973 the amendment developed new residential care services, such as short stay or day care services. The Health and Medical Service Act for the Aged of 1982 started for those who were 70 years old and older, and in 1990 the amendment shifted from

Chapter 6   International Migration, Wellness, and Social Policies in the United States, Sweden, and Japan   151

institutional care to residential care conducted by municipalities.

Long-Term Care Insurance was instituted in 2000 in which the main mission was to support older citizens so that they could live independently in communities. With this insurance, most of older adults could access comprehensive health care and social services by choosing from hospitals, nursing homes, and group homes (Ministry of Health, Labor, and Welfare, 2012a, 2012b). In 2011 Long-Term Care Insurance was amended to provide more sensitive community-based health and social services, particularly for those with early dementia.

Hence, it should be suggested challenges of social policy for elderly care in Japan such as financial cost effectiveness of national health care insurance and long-term care insurance, and the insufficient number of care facilities that may extend the duration of at-home caregiving by family members and lead to serious burdens.

CHINESE MIGRATION AND HEALTHY AGING

This section will examine Chinese domestic and international migration and healthy aging among older adults and older immigrants of Chinese and other ethnic groups in China, the United States, Sweden, and Japan. The author first will focus on Chinese domestic and international migration and healthy aging among older adults and older immigrants in China.

China

Chen & Liu (2012) reported that physical health and well-being of grandparents who lived with grandchildren and cared for grandchildren were associated with household income, resident regions, children's

152   Part 3   Future Directions

migration, statuses of grandparents (i.e., paternal or maternal grandparents), and levels of care. Paternal grandparents who provided a lower level of care for grandchildren, had higher household income, received financial support from migrated adult children, and lived in urban areas showed better self-rated health than their counterparts in rural areas.

Cong & Silverstein (2011) suggested elderly parents who have higher depressive symptoms indicated lower financial, instrumental, and emotional support from sons since the patrilineal family system distinguishes sons from daughters concerning their role in supporting elderly parents' social networks in rural China. Guo, Chi, & Silverstein (2011) also noted that a greater distance between elderly parents and adult children were associated with their closer relationships, and that having more children and greater variability in distance between elderly parents and adult children increased father's differentiation due to the context of son-preference and out-migration in rural China. These findings imply that adult children's large-scale migration have affected traditional familism norms, intergenerational support, and physical and mental health among older adults in China.

The United States

In the United States, Chinese international migration and healthy aging have closely linked among older adults and older immigrants. Dong, Chang, Wong, & Simon (2012) analyzed depression among older Chinese immigrants in Chicago and found higher depressive symptoms on resulted from worsening physical health, financial strains, family conflicts, and societal conflicts (i.e., acculturation stress, social isolation, and difficulties with the health system). Specifically, intergenerational gaps endorsed family

Chapter 6 International Migration, Wellness, and Social Policies in the United States, Sweden, and Japan   153

conflicts in which older adults had higher expectations to be taken care of by younger generations than children, and children sometimes neglected elderly parents because of their longer hard working hours as well as differences in habits and lifestyle choices.

However, comparing Chinese immigrants in the United States with native-born Chinese living in China, Wu, Chi, Plassman, & Guo (2010) reported that older Chinese Americans had a significantly lower level of depressive symptoms than older Chinese. Arthritis and back or neck problems were associated with a higher level of depressive symptoms among Chinese Americans, whereas problems in walking were associated with depression among older Chinese. An appropriate understanding of depression is pivotal to provide culturally competent health care and social services for these populations (Wu, Chi, Plassman, & Guo, 2010). Also, the association between stronger social network and better self-reported health is affected by additional factors such as socioeconomic status, health behaviors, and access to health care (Wu, Guo, Chi, & Plassman, 2011).

Sweden

In terms of international migration to Sweden and healthy aging among older adults and older immigrants, Silviera, Skoog, Sundth, Allebeck, & Steen (2002) noted that older immigrants, indicated lower levels of physical health, economic status, and satisfaction with family life than did older native-born Swedes. From the Survey of Health, Aging and Retirement in Europe (SHARE), which included 11 European countries, older immigrants living in Switzerland, Denmark, the Netherlands, and Sweden were more likely to have lower levels of activities of daily living (ADL) and instrumental activities of daily living (IADL) than other countries, and

154   Part 3   Future Directions

Sweden had the lowest self-reported health (Sole-Auro & Crimmins, 2008).

As Leao, Sundquist, Johansson, & Sundquist (2009) suggested, health care providers and policy makers need to pay special attention to health care for immigrants, in particular first generation immigrants of advanced age who have lived less than 15 years in Sweden, as they reported poorer self-rated health than their counterparts.

Japan

Healthy aging research on older native-born adults and older immigrants has underdeveloped in Japan. Tajima (2003) described Chinese immigrants who had moved from Mainland China and Taiwan in the decades after China's Reform and Open Door Policy of 1978. These immigrants expanded their ethnic networks in urban regions and faced challenges of finding jobs and housing because of language barriers and discrimination. Onishi (2001) noted that language proficiency, work environment, financial status, and separation from their home countries were significant stressors among South Eastern Asian immigrants who had lived in Japan less than five years, while difficulties in advanced interpersonal skills and unfamiliarity with Japanese traditional family customs were dominant stressors among those who had lived in Japan more than five years.

Schwingel et al. (2007) reported that Japanese Brazilians living in San Paulo had a lower level of high-density lipoprotein cholesterol (HDL-cholesterol) than native-born Japanese and Japanese Brazilians living in Japan in which cardiovascular diseases are affected by genetic and environmental factors. Triglycerides, waist circumference, LDL-cholesterol, meat intake, stress, and smoking were negatively associated with HDL-cholesterol, while total cholesterol, fish intake, and physical activity were

Chapter 6   International Migration, Wellness, and Social Policies in the United States, Sweden, and Japan   155

positively associated with it. These are considered as environmental factors in which immigrants living in Brazil, a diverse immigrant country, may have lower stress than native-born Japanese and immigrants living in Japan, which is a homogeneous country and is not open to diversity. As Kawamura (2009) noted, development of multicultural caregiving is essential for older Chinese and Korean immigrants who had been forced to move to Japan before and during World War Two.

POLICY IMPLICATIONS OF INTERNATIONAL MIGRATION AND WELLNESS

This section will propose policy implications of international migration and wellness among older Chinese immigrants in China, the United States, Sweden, and Japan. In Sweden, all immigrants can access universal health care services regardless of working duration, medical history, and family status. In the United States, if older immigrants are documented as legal residents at least five years, they are eligible for Medicare. However, if they did not pay taxes for Medicare for ten years, they have to pay a premium every month to keep Medicare enrollment. Also, if they are eligible for Medicaid, they dually have Medicare and Medicaid. However, as health care costs are extremely expensive in the United States, Medicare as well as Medicaid sometimes do not cover all expenses. The U.S. health policies are particularly complicated, and it is hard for older Chinese immigrants and their families to understand accessibility to health services (Dong, Chang, Wong, & Simon, 2012).

In Japan, if they are documented as legal residents or have Japanese citizenship, they are eligible for National Health Insurance. If they have dementia and/or serious declines of activities of daily living (ADL), they are eligible for Long-Term Care Insurance after assessment teams have qualified them. If they are dependents of their children's families, their children must pay the premium of their company's health insurance for themselves and dependents. However, as seen in the recent economic recession, if their children lose full-time jobs and their company's health insurance, they face difficulties in paying both the premium of National Health Insurance and Long-Term Care Insurance.

As aging is a natural process among human beings, elderly care is considered a human right (Edebalk, 2010) and should be independent from any politics and economics (Barr, 2010). Each country may examine more cost effectiveness of social policy not only for its aging population but also for younger generations. Also, culturally-generationally-linguistically sensitive health services for older Chinese immigrants should be developed in the United States, Sweden, and Japan. As another policy implication, reflecting the highest international migration and transient migrant patterns, international organizations such as the United Nations and OECD, should examine international social policies for elderly care and its global governance. Because of increasing populations and health care costs among industrialized countries, each country as well as international organization should examine cost effective universal social policy for elderly care.

Hopefully, all citizens and immigrants can live independently in communities as long as possible and will actualize social inclusion in communities with balanced social policies and health care systems in the near future. All generations will respectfully exchange social supports beyond family in our global super aging societies.

ACKNOWLEDGMENTS

This study was funded by the Residential Faculty Fellowship of the Institute of East Asian Studies at the University of California at Berkeley and was partly presented at the Residential Faculty Fellowship Awardee Seminar at the University of California at Berkeley. The author wishes thank you for Dr. Winston Tseng, who is a commentator at the workshop. The author also appreciates Dr. Andrew E. Scharlach as a chair and commentator at the workshop.

REFERENCES

Baar, D.A. (2010). *Introduction to U.S. health policy: The organization, financing, and delivery of health care in America (3 rd ed.).* Baltimore: Johns Hopkins University Press.

Burgess, A.M., & Burgess, C.G. (2006). Ageing-in-place: Present realities and future directions. *Forum on Public Policy: A Journal of the Oxford Round Table.* Retrieved November 2, 2011 from http://www.forumonpublicpolicy.com/archive07/burgess.pdf

Chen, F., & Liu, G. (2012). The health implications of grandparents caring for grandchildren in China. *The Journals of Gerontology Series B: Psychological Sciences and Social Sciences, 67*(1), 99-112.

China National Committee on Aging (2011). *The twelfth five-year plan for aging policy in Shanghai.* Retrieved June 3, 2011 from http://www.yinlingguanai.org/2011/0509/240.html (in Chinese).

Cong, Z., & Silverstein, M. (2011). Parents' depressive symptoms and support from sons and daughters in rural China. *International Journal of Social Welfare, 20,* S4-S17.

Dong, X., Chang, E.-S., Wong, E., & Simon, M. (2012). The perceptions, social determinants, and negative health outcomes associated with depressive symptoms among U.S. Chinese older adults. *Gerontologist, 52*(5), 650-663.

158   Part 3   Future Directions

Edebalk, P.G. (2010). Ways of funding and organizing elderly care in Sweden, In T. Bengtsson (Ed.) *Population ageing: A threat to welfare state?* (pp.65-80). New York: Springer.

Eggleston, K. (2012). Health care for 1.3 billion. *Working paper series on health and demographic change in the Asia-Pacific.* Stanford, CA: Walter H. Shorenstein Asia-Pacific Research Center, Stanford University.

Guo, M., Chi, I., & Silverstein, M. (2011). Family as a context: The influence of family composition and family geographic dispersion on intergenerational relationships among Chinese elderly. *International Journal of Social Welfare, 20,* S18-S29.

Hoshino, K. (2012a). *Social policy and healthy aging among older Chinese immigrants in the United States, Sweden, and Japan.* Paper presented at the Residential Faculty Fellowship Awardee Seminar in the Institute of East Asian Studies at the University of California at Berkeley (Berkeley, CA).

Hoshino, K. (2012b). Sociocultural support model for healthy aging: Perspectives from the United States, Sweden, and Japan. In A.E. Scharlach & K. Hoshino (Eds.) *Healthy aging in sociocultural contexts* (pp.85-96). New York: Routledge.

Hoshino, K. (2012c). Healthy aging and policy implications for older immigrants in Japan. In A.E. Scharlach & K. Hoshino (Eds.) *Healthy aging in sociocultural contexts* (pp.72-81). New York: Routledge.

Kawamura, C. (2009). *Imin seisaku heno apurochi [Approach to immigration policy].* Tokyo: Akashi Shoten.

Kinsella, K., & He, W. (2009). *An aging world: 2008.* International population reports. Washington, DC: U.S. Census Bureau.

Konkurrendverket (2007). *Oka Konsumentnyttan inom vard och omsorg-forslag for konkurrens och okat foretagande.* Konkurrensverkets rapportserie 2007 (in Swedish).

Leao, T.S., Sundquist, J., Johansson, S.-E., & Sundquist, K. (2009). The influence of age at migration and length of residence on self-rated health among Swedish immigrants: A cross-sectional study. *Ethnicity & Health, 14*(1), 93-105.

Liang, H.C. (1995). *The health management of the aged in China.* Paper presented at the 5 th Asia Oceania Regional Congress of Gerontology (Hong Kong).

Lou, V.W., & Gui, S. (2011). Family caregiving and impact on caregiver mental health: A study in Shanghai. In Chen, S. & Powell, J.L. (Eds.) *Aging in China:*

Implications to social policy of a changing economic state (pp.187-207). New York: Springer.

Ministry of Health, Labor, and Welfare. (2012a). *Long-Term Care Insurance and its future direction.* Tokyo: Ministry of Health, Labor, and Welfare. Retrieved January 15, 2012 from http://www.mhlw.go.jp/topics/kaigo/gaiyo/.

Ministry of Health, Labor, and Welfare. (2012b).*The 2011 annual white report on health, labor, and welfare.* Tokyo: Ministry of Health, Labor, and Welfare.

Naerssen, T.V., Spaan, E., & Zoomers, A. (Eds.) (2008) *Global migration and development.* New York: Routledge.

Nakagawa, T., & Gondo, Y. (2012). Health care system and policy implications for older adults in Japan. In A.E. Scharlach & K. Hoshino (Eds.) *Healthy aging in sociocultural contexts* (pp.53-61). New York: Routledge.

National Bureau of Statistics of China (2011). China statistics yearbook 2011. Retrieved June 3, 2011 from http://www.stats.gov.cn/tjsj/ndsj/2010/indexch. htm.

National News Office of People's Republic of China (2006). Press release: The development of China's undertakings for the aged.

Organisation for Economic Co-operation and Development (2009). *The future of international migration to OECD countries.* Paris: OECD.

Organization for Economic Co-operation and Development (2010). *International migration outlook.* Paris: OECD.

Onishi, A. (2001). "Gaikokujin rodosha" no sutoresu taisho to sogo enjyo soshiki no yakuwari [Stress coping of "foreign workers" and role of mutual help organization]. *Japanese Journal of Community Psychology, 4*(2), 107-118.

Patient Protection and Affordable Care Act of 2010 (2010). H.R. 3590; Pub.L. 111-148; 124 Stat. 119-1024. 111 th Congress; March 23, 2010.

Rowe, J.W., & Kahn, R.L. (1987). Human aging: Usual and successful. *Science, 237,* 143-149.

Rowe, J.W., & Kahn, R.L. (1988). *Successful aging.* New York: Pantheon.

Satariano, W.A. (2006). *Epidemiology of aging: An ecological approach.* Sudbury, MA: Jones and Barlett.

Satariano, W.A. (2012). Healthy aging in the U.S. In A.E. Scharlach & K. Hoshino (Eds.) *Healthy aging in sociocultural contexts* (pp.14-21). New York: Routledge.

160　　Part 3　Future Directions

Scharlach, A. E., & Hoshino, K. (2012). Conclusion. In A.E. Scharlach & K. Hoshino (Eds.) *Healthy aging in sociocultural contexts* (pp.96-105). New York: Routledge.

Schwingel, A., Nakata, Y., Ito, L.S., Chodzko-Zajko, W.J., Shigematsu, R., Erb, C.T., Souza, S.M., Oba-Shinjo, S.M., Matuo, T., Marie, S.K.N., & Tanaka, K. (2007). Lower HDL-cholesterol among healthy middle-aged Japanese-Brazilians in San Paulo compared to Natives and Japanese-Brazilians in Japan. *European Journal of Epidemiology, 22*, 33-42.

Shanghai Committee on Aging (2006). The eleventh five-year plan for aging policy in Shanghai. Retrieved June 3, 2011 from http://www.shmzj-gov.cn/gb/shmzj/node8/node15/node55/node231/node263/userobject1ai22366.html (in Chinese).

Silviera, E., Skoog, I., Sundth, V., Allebeck, P., & Steen, B. (2002). Health and well-being among 70 years old migrants living in Sweden: Results from the H70 gerontological and geriatric population studies of Goteborg. *Social Psychiatry and Psychiatric Epidemiology, 37*, 13-22.

Socialstyrelsen (2007).*Vard och omsorg om alder.* Lagesrapport 2006. (in Swedish).

Sole-Auro, A., & Crimmins, E.M. (2008). Health of immigrants in European countries. *International Migration Review, 42*(4), 861-876.

Steering Committee of the National People's Congress of People's Republic of China (1996). *People's Republic of China Law on the Protection of the Rights and Interests of Older People.* Retrieved June 3, 2011 from http://fss.mca.gov.cn/article/lnrfl/zcfg/200903/20090300027331.shtml (in Chinese).

Tajima, J. (2003). Chinese newcomers in the global city Tokyo: Social networks and settlement tendencies. *International Journal of Japanese Sociology, 12*, 68-78.

Thuno, M. (2007). *Beyond Chinatown: New Chinese migration and the global expansion of China.* Copenhagen: Nordic Institute of Asian Studies Press.

U.S. Census Bureau (2011). *2011 national population projections.* Washington, DC: U.S. Census Bureau Population Division.

World Bank (2015). *The World Bank open data.* Retrieved November 6, 2015 from http://data.world-bank.org/indicator/SP.POP.65UP.TO.ZS.

Wu, B., Chi, I., Plassman, B.L., & Guo, M. (2010). Depressive symptoms and health problems among Chinese immigrant elders in the US and Chinese elders in China. *Aging & Mental Health, 14*(6), 695-704.

Wu, B., Guo, M., Chi, I.,& Plassman, B.L. (2011). Social network and health: A comparison of Chinese older adults in Shanghai and elderly immigrants in Boston. *International Journal of Social Welfare, 20*, S59-S71.

Zhang, N.J., Guo, M., & Zheng, X. (2012). China: Awaking giant developing solutions to population aging. *Gerontologist, 52*(5), 589-596.

Chapter 7 Conclusions

Kazumi Hoshino

INTERNATIONAL MIGRATION AND WELLNESS INNOVATION

This book has examined international migration and wellness innovation in the United States, Sweden, and Japan, which reflect global demographic changes, including the low fertility rates, declining labor forces, longevity, and increasing diversity. Wellness is optimal physical, mental and emotional well-being and emphasizes personal responsibility for making the lifestyle choices and self-care decisions that will improve the quality of one's life (Berkeley Wellness.com, 2015). Although health is defined as a state of complete physical, mental, and social well-being, and not merely the absence of diseases (WHO, 2015), wellness transcends the definition of health and leads to multidimensional perspectives. Wellness consists of eight dimensions: emotional, social, environmental, financial, intellectual, occupational, physical, and spiritual (Smarbrick, 2006). Learning about the eight dimensions of wellness will help people choose how to pursue wellness in their daily lives (SAMHSA, 2015).

The author analyzed associations between international migration and wellness, in particular emotional and social dimensions. Emotional dimension refers to coping effectively with life and creating satisfying relationships, while social dimension is defined as developing a sense of connection, belonging, and a well-developed support system. In this publication, the author focused on cultural identity and intergenerational support and social policies of healthy aging among older adults in terms of social dimension. Emotional dimension was analyzed from the perspectives of intergenerational relationships. It is essential to clarify how international migration may affect wellness among immigrants in the United States, Sweden, and Japan in terms of social dimension (i.e., cultural identity, intergenerational support, and social policies of elderly health care and social services) and emotional dimension (i.e., intergenerational relationships), while immigrants may try to maintain its consistency and handle changes in their lives as they transition from their home countries to their new countries.

CULTURAL INDENTITY, INTERGENERATIONAL RELATIONSHIPS, AND INTERGENERATIONAL SUPPORT IN THE UNITED STATES AND SWEDEN

In chapter 1, the authors examined commonalities and differences in cultural identity and intergenerational relationships from the perspectives of Chinese Americans, Japanese Americans, and Peruvian Americans of the first generation adult immigrants in the United States and proposed a new Model of Cultural Identity, Intergenerational Relationships, and Intergenerational Support, based on a content analysis in chapter 2. The model indicated that cultural identity, intergenerational support, and intergenerational relationships may be affected by demographic variables, including age, gender, education, current job, socioeconomic status, language proficiency, immigrant generation, and migration patterns. Diversity, social values such as political systems and health care policies, generational reciprocity, and familism norms influenced cultural identity and were also related to intergenerational support. Moreover, cultural identity and intergenerational support associated with intergenerational relationships between children, adults, and elderly parents.

Chapter 3 analyzed social policies of social inclusion and mental health in terms of cultural identity, intergenerational support, and intergenerational relationships among diverse immigrants in Sweden. As policy implications, policymakers, as well as health care professionals, need to develop culturally competent health care services which correspond to support needs among diverse ethnic populations. Also, international organizations such as the European Union should have information on the area of origin of immigrants and how that differs across countries in terms of the database from an international perspective. In addition, global migration network of health care professionals should have possibilities to support immigrants in order to minimize adversity and to promote their healthy lifespan development.

ETHNIC INDENTITY, INTERGENARATIONAL SUPPORT, AND PSYCHOSOCIAL DEVLOPMENT IN JAPAN

In chapter 4, the author developed the Multigroup Ethnic Identity Measure-Revised Japanese Version and identified associations between ethnic identity, intergenerational support, and psychosocial development among younger adults and older adults in Japan in chapter 5. Identity was significant and positively associated with Exploration and Commitment of ethnic identity among older adults, although identity was not significantly

166   Part 3 Future Directions

associated with ethnic identity among younger adults. Generativity had significant and positive associations with Exploration among younger adults and older adults. Of gerotranscendence, only the Cosmic Dimension was significant and positively associated with Exploration and Commitment among younger adults and older adults. In terms of intergenerational support, only receiving support from younger generations had significant and positive association with Commitment among older adults. The Japanese older adults may be promoted commitment to ethnic identity in terms of receiving support from younger generations, while younger adults may have less opportunity to struggle with ethnic identity.

INTERNATIONAL MIGRATION AND WELLNESS IN THE UNITED STATES, SWEDEN, AND JAPAN

The author conducted an international comparative research on healthy aging as wellness among older adults and social policies of elderly care in the United States, Sweden, and Japan in terms of Chinese migration to the three countries and in their home country in chapter 6. Since elderly care is considered a human right (Edebalk, 2010), it should be independent from any politics and economics (Barr, 2010). Each country should propose more cost effectiveness of social policy and culturally competent health services. Also, international organizations such as the United Nations should examine international elderly care policies and its global governance. Each nation and international organizations should consider cost effective universal social policy for elderly care due to increasing older populations and health care costs among industrialized countries.

WELLNESS INNOVATION AND MULTICULCURAL SUPPORT

Wellness promotion and improvement among immigrants and refugees are essential in their transitions from their home countries to their immigrated countries, and also the introduction act and the orientation program are necessary because they are vulnerable at the forefront of international migration. Regeringskansliet (The Swedish Ministry of Integration and Gender Equality, 2010) reformed the introduction policy which facilitates the introduction of newly arrived immigrants into working and community lives, by strengthening the personal incentives to take up work and take an active part in employment preparatory activities. The civic orientation is an obligatory part of the introduction for newly arrived immigrants highlights the importance of human rights and fundamental democratic values as well as the Individual's rights and obligations. The program of the civic orientation consists of eight areas: Coming to Sweden; Living in Sweden; Supporting yourself and developing in Sweden; The rights and obligations of the individual; Starting a family and living with children in Sweden; Having influence in Sweden; Caring for your health in Sweden; and Growing old in Sweden. The municipalities are obliged to offer newly arrived immigrants a minimum of 60 hours of civic orientation.

In this final section, the author demonstrates a Multidisciplinary and Multicultural Support Model for Immigrants (Figure 7-1, Hoshino, 2016) as a policy implication of international migration and wellness innovation, by reviewing relevant policies (Swedish Institute, 2012; Migrationsverket, 2010; Ministry of Health, Labour, and Welfare, 2012; Cabinet Office, 2003, 2007a, 2007b). This model represents support for immigrants in their processes, while they enter into host countries, adjust to new communities, and

168   Part 3   Future Directions

collaborate with international societies. The Comprehensive Multicultural Support Center provides multidisciplinary support for immigrants, refugees, migrant workers, and international students, by collaborating with various professionals of municipalities, education, health care, social welfare, law, ethnic organizations, religious associations, and key persons in communities. The coordinators, such as psychologists and/or other professionals, integrates multidisciplinary collaboration and coordinates appropriate multicultural support in terms of the network conference. Interpreters are available for immigrants in all processes upon their entry into new countries.

The Comprehensive Multicultural Support Center for Immigrants consists of four functions: Education, Research, Counseling Services, and Coordination (Table 7-1, Hoshino, 2016). Education includes Educational programs for immigrants: Educational programs on culture, social life, health care, social welfare, and basic laws; Language programs on immigrants' first language, second language, and English; School education assistant programs for immigrants' children and adolescents; Employment support programs; and Educational programs on financial aid policies for low-income people. Also, Education offers Educational programs for native-born nationals: Global professional internships for undergraduate and graduate students; and Global lifelong educational programs for multicultural professionals.

Research conducts international studies as well as local studies: Research on international collaborations of multidisciplinary and multicultural support; Research on evaluation of education; Research on evaluation of counseling services; and Research on evaluation of coordination. Counseling Services offer Law counseling services, Health care counseling services, Psychological counseling services, and Social welfare counseling services for immigrants. Coordination coordinates the three services: Network conference of multidisciplinary and multicultural support for professionals; Coordination of collaboration with professionals such as researchers and practitioners of law, medicine, education, health care, social welfare, and psychology; and Referral to other professional facilities of specific cases such as alcohol dependence and substance abuse and urgent cases, including child abuse, elderly abuse, and domestic violence.

The model embraces administrative conferences in the two levels to facilitate each professional support for immigrants and collaborations in the network: Practitioners' Conference; and Senior Officials' Conference. The Practitioners' Conference examines missions and methods of immigrant support, urgent interventions, and roles of relevant facilities. The Senior Officials' Conference periodically evaluates all cases of the immigrants requiring protection and revises support missions and methods. The Senior Officials' Conference also advocates immigrant support in communities and evaluates the network system as a whole.

Multicultural support for immigrants should be based on culturally competent services and should correspond to their linguistic understanding. Wellness promotion will expand multidimensional perspectives of human development and will embrace diversity in international societies, as well as local communities. Although this book has examined emotional dimension in terms of intergenerational relationships as well as social dimension with regard to cultural identity, intergenerational support, and social policies for elderly care, future research should deal with all dimensions. Collaborations with other professionals and translational research in natural sciences and

170   Part 3   Future Directions

Immigration Processes	Professional Institutes and Network Conference of Multidisciplinary and Multicultural Support on Legal Issues

Entry Permit	**National Government: Ministry of Law, Ministry of Immigration**

Foreign Resident
Registration

Network Conference of Multidisciplinary and Multicultural Support

Senior Officials' Conference
· Examination of Cases with Protection
· Evaluation of the Support System

|

Practitioners' Conference
· Discussion of the Mission and Methods
· Examination of Each Role of Professionals

Social and
Cultural
Adjustment in
New Countries

Comprehensive Multicultural Support Center for Immigrants

Coordinators: Psychologists and Professionals

· Education for Immigrants and Native-Born
  Nationals
· Research on International Collaboration and
  Evaluation of Services
· Counseling Services on Law, Health, Social
  Welfare, and Psychology
· Coordination of Network Conference and
  Professional Collaboration

Crime Prevention

Local Government/Municipalities
· Information of Health Care
  and Social Welfare Services
· Information of Financial Aids
  for Low Income Population
· Information of Social Security
· Second Language Programs

Community-Based Organizations
· Cultural Information of Home
  Countries and New Countries
· Consultation on Access and
  Barriers of Law, Health Care,
  and Social Welfare Services
· Interpretation and Translation

Chapter 7   Conclusions   171

		Immigrants

If Crime Occur

Police
· Arrest
· Crime Victims Support

Religious Associations
· Spiritual Support
· Faith

During Trial

Public Prosecutors Offices
· Indictment
· Crime Victims Support

Hospitals/Clinics
· Medical Treatment
· Diagnosis

Legal Support Centers
· Appointed Court Counsel
· Civil Legal Aid
· Crime Victims Support

Psychological Clinics
· Clinical Assessment
· Counseling Services
· Psychological Community
   Support

Bar Associations
· Litigation Support
· Judicial Cost Support
· Crime Victims Support

Social Welfare Facilities
· Social Welfare Services
· Community Support

Court
· Trial
· Judgement

Schools/Universities
· School Education
· Lifelong Learning

Social Adjustment
in Communities
If Found Not Guilty

Key Persons in Communities
· Understanding of Immigrants' Needs
· Exploration of Service Barriers

Social Adjustment
in Communities
After Release from
Prison, If Found Guilty
Collaboration with
International Societies

**Figure 7-1 A Model of Multidisciplinary and Multicultural Support
for Immigrants (Hoshino, 2016)**

172   Part 3   Future Directions

Table 7-1 Functions of the Comprehensive Multicultural Support Center (Hoshino, 2016)

Functions

1. Education
1) Educational programs for immigrants
(1) Educational programs on culture, social life, health care, social welfare, and basic laws
(2) Language learning programs of immigrants' original languages, second languages, and English
(3) School education assistant programs for immigrant children and adolescents
(4) Employment support programs
(5) Educational programs on policies of financial aids for low-income people

2) Educational programs for native-born nationals
(1) Global professional internships for undergraduate and graduate students
(2) Global lifelong educational programs for multicultural professionals

2. Research
1) Research on international collaborations of multidisciplinary and multicultural support
2) Research on evaluation of education
3) Research on evaluation of clinical services
4) Research on evaluation of coordination

3. Counseling services
1) Law counseling services for immigrants
2) Health care counseling services for immigrants
3) Psychological counseling services for immigrants
4) Social welfare counseling services for immigrants

4. Coordination
1) Network conference of multidisciplinary and multicultural support professionals
2) Coordination of collaboration with professionals such as researchers and practitioners of law, medicine, education, health care, social welfare, and psychology
3) Referral to professional facilities of specific cases such as alcohol dependence and substance abuse and urgent cases, including abuse and domestic violence

Chapter 7　Conclusions　173

social sciences are particularly important to facilitate appropriate multicultural support for international migration and wellness innovation.

ACKNOWLEDGMENTS

The author wishes to thank the Editorial Committee of Compilation and Documentation on Refugees and Migrants Quarterly for their permission of reprinting the table and the figure for this book. This study was funded by the Association of Japanese Clinical Psychology.

REFERENCES

Baar, D.A. (2010). *Introduction to U.S. health policy: The organization, financing, and delivery of health care in America (3rd ed.).* Baltimore: Johns Hopkins University Press.

Berkeley Wellness.com (2015). What is wellness? Retrieved July 12, 2015 from http://www.berkeleywellness.com/about-us

Cabinet Office (2003). Research report on domestic violence for female partners, Tokyo: Cabinet Office.

Cabinet Office (2007a). A handbook model of support for crime victims, Tokyo: Cabinet Office.

Cabinet Office (2007b). Final report on collaborative support, Tokyo: Cabinet Office.

Edebalk, P.G. (2010). Ways of funding and organizing elderly care in Sweden, In T. Bengtsson (Ed.) *Population ageing: A threat to welfare state?* (pp.65-80). New York: Springer.

Hoshino, K. (2016). Multidisciplinary and Multicultural Support Model for Immigrants on Legal Issues, *Compilation and Documentation on Refugees and Migrants Quarterly* (in press).

Migrationsverket (2010). Residence permits granted and registered rights of residence 2010, Stockholm: Migrationsverket.

Ministry of Health, Labour, and Welfare (2012). Case report of associations of

174　Part 3　Future Directions

children with protection, Tokyo: Ministry of Health, Labour, and Welfare.

Regeringskansliet (2010). New policy for the introduction of newly arrived immigrants in Sweden. Stockholm: Regeringskansliet.

Substance Abuse and Mental Health Services Administration (2015). SAMHSA Wellness Initiative. Retrieved July 12, 2015 from http://www.samhsa.gov/wellness-initiative

Smarbrick, M. (2006). A Wellness Approach, *Psychiatric Rehabilitation Journal*, *29*(4), 311-314.

Swedish Institute (2012). Facts about Sweden: Disability Policy. Stockholm: Swedish Institute.

World Health Organization (2015). Definition of health. Retrieved June 28, 2015 from http://www.who.int

Appendix

Appendix 1

Informed Consent Form of Cultural Identity and Intergenerational Relationships among Diverse Adults in the United States (Chapters 1 and 2)

CONSENT TO PARTICIPATE IN A RESEARCH STUDY

TITLE OF STUDY: Cultural Beliefs and Family Intergenerational Relationships among Culturally Diverse Adults

INVESTIGATORS:

Winston Tseng, Ph.D.
School of Public Health
University of California, Berkeley
Phone: (   )

Kazumi Hoshino, Ph.D.
School of Public Health
University of California, Berkeley
Phone: (   )

Introduction and Purpose:

My name is Dr. Hoshino and I'm a visiting scholar at the University of California, Berkeley working with my faculty sponsor, Dr. Tseng, in the School of Public Health. I would like to invite you to take part in this research study, which examines cultural beliefs and family intergenerational relationships among Japanese, Chinese, and Hispanic descendants between the ages 40-59 years old. We want to know whether there are differences among cultural groups. We will use what we learn to find ways to promote cultural identity and to improve intergenerational relationships across multicultural adult populations.

PROCEDURES: If you agree to take part in this research study, a member of the research team will interview you in person at a time and place convenient to you or the UC Berkeley, School of Public Health office. Just before the interview starts, we will ask you to complete a short demographic survey about yourself. During the interview, we will ask you some questions about your perspectives on cultural beliefs and family relationships, and the perspectives of your children and older parents. The interview will last up to 90 minutes. With your permission, we will make sound recordings of the interview. After the interview, we will type up the interview discussion.

ALTERNATIVE: You can choose not to take part in the study. You may also choose to stop being in the study at any time. There will be no penalty to you.

RISKS: The risks are minimal. As with all research, there is a chance that confidentiality could be compromised; however, we are taking precautions to minimize this risk. Some of the questions about cultural identity and perspectives of family members may be sensitive to you. You have the right to refuse to answer any questions and you can stop the interview at any time.

BENEFITS: Although you will not benefit directly from participating in this research, the information you provide may help improve understanding about cultural beliefs and intergenerational relationships among Japanese, Chinese, and Hispanic families.

CONFIDENTIALITY: Your study data will be handled as confidentially as possible. If results of this study are published or presented, individual names and other personally identifiable information will not be used. Data will be coded and will never be associated with personally identifiable information, only a number will be used to identify your record. Your record, with this number, will only be recorded on the participant log. This participant log will be kept in a locked file cabinet and/or a password protected computer file where it cannot be accessed by anyone who is not a member of the research team.

COSTS/COMPENSATION: There is no cost to you beyond the time and efforts required to participate in the interview and complete the survey. You will be paid $25 for your participation even if you do not fully complete the interview.

RIGHT TO REFUSE OR WITHDRAW: Participation in research is completely voluntary. You are free to decline to take part in the project. You can decline to answer any questions and are free to stop taking part in the project at any time. Whether or not you choose to participate in the research and whether or not you choose to answer a question or continue participating in the project, there will be no penalty to you or loss of benefits to which you are otherwise entitled.

QUESTIONS: If you have any questions about this research, please feel free to contact me. I can be reached at (Phone Number) or (Email Address).

If you have any questions about your rights or treatment as a research participant in this study, please contact the University of California at Berkeley's Committee for Protection of Human Subjects at (Phone Number) or (Email Address).

WRITTEN CONSENT: Your signature below indicates that you have given consent to volunteer as a research subject and that you have read and understood the information provided above.

Appendix   179

Participant Name:_____

Signature of Participant_____

Date_____

The purpose of the study has been explained to me to my satisfaction. I have had the opportunity to ask questions and to have my questions answered. I voluntarily agree to participate in this research study.

180

Appendix 2

Demographic Form of Cultural Identity and Intergenerational Relationships (Chapters 1 and 2)

Case #:_____
Participant ID:_____
Interview Date (mm/dd/yyyy):_____
Length of Interview (hh:mm):_____
Interview Location:_____
Interviewer Name:_____

DEMOGRAPHIC SURVEY

We would like to know more about you. Please circle the most appropriate answer or provide a written response.

1. Respondent Gender: 1) male   2) female

2. What country were you born?
   1) The United States   2) Peru   3) China   4) Taiwan   5) Japan
   6) Other: Please specify: _____

3. At what age did you first migrate to the United States? _____

4. How old are you? _____years

5. What is your marital status?
   1) Single   2) Married   3) Separated   4) Widowed   5)Divorced

6. Do you have children?
   1) Yes → a. How many children do you have? How many? _____
            b. How frequently do you have contact with your children?
               Please specify: _____
   2) No children

7. Do you have any grandchildren?
   1) Yes → a. How many grandchildren do you have? How many? _____
            b. How frequently do you have contact with your grandchildren?
               Please specify: _____
   2) No grandchildren

Appendix   181

8. How many years of education did you complete? _____ years

9. What is your current occupation?
   1) Homemaker   2) Caregiver   3) Construction   4) Service   5) Clerical
   6) Business   7) Professional   8) Retired   9) Unemployed
   10) Other: Please specify: _____

10. Who do you currently live with? (Please select ALL that apply.)
   1) Alone   2) Spouse/Partner   3) Children   4) Grandchildren
   5) Parents   6) Relatives   7) Others (Please specify:_____)
   For how many months or years have you been in this living arrangement? ____

11. What was your family household income last year?
   1) -$19,999   2) $20,000-$39,999   3) $40,000-$59,999
   4) $60,000-$79,999   5) $80,000-$99,999   6) ≥ $100,000

12. Since you immigrated to the U.S. how many times have you migrated back and
   forth to your country of origin?
   1) Less than 3 times   2) 3-6 times   3) 6-9 times   4) More than 9 times

13. What country was your father born in?
   1) The United States   2) Peru   3) China   4) Taiwan   5) Japan
   6) Other: Please specify: _____

14. What country was your mother born?
   1) The United States   2) Peru   3) China   4) Taiwan   5) Japan
   6) Other: Please specify: _____

15. What country does your father currently live in?
   1) The United States   2) Peru   3) China   4) Taiwan   5) Japan
   6) Other: Please specify: _____

16. What country does your mother currently live in?
   1) The United States   2) Peru   3) China   4) Taiwan   5) Japan
   6) Other: Please specify: _____

17. The following questions refer to your language use, please circle the most appropriate
   response.

17a. What is your language of origin?
　　　　　　1) Japanese　　2) Cantonese　　3) Mandarin　　4) Spanish
　　　　　　5) Other: Please Specify: _____

17b. In general, what language(s) do you prefer to use when reading and speaking?
　　　1=[Language of origin] Only
　　　2=[Language of origin] Better than English
　　　3=Both Equally
　　　4=English Better than [Language of origin]
　　　5=English Only

17c. What language(s) do you usually speak at home?
　　　1=[Language of origin] Only
　　　2=[Language of origin] Better than English
　　　3=Both Equally
　　　4=English Better than [Language of origin]
　　　5=English Only

17d. In which language(s) do you usually use when thinking?
　　　1=[Language of origin] Only
　　　2=[Language of origin] Better than English
　　　3=Both Equally
　　　4=English Better than [Language of origin]
　　　5=English Only

17e. What language(s) do you usually speak with your friends?
　　　1=[Language of origin] Only
　　　2=[Language of origin] Better than English
　　　3=Both Equally
　　　4=English Better than [Language of origin]
　　　5=English Only

17f. What was the language you used as a child?
　　　1=[Language of origin] Only
　　　2=[Language of origin] Better than English
　　　3=Both Equally
　　　4=English Better than [Language of origin]
　　　5=English Only

Thank you for your participation.

Appendix   183

Appendix 3

Interview Protocol of Cultural Identity and Intergenerational Relationships (Chapters 1 and 2)

Case #:_____

Participant ID:_____

Interview Date (mm/dd/yyyy):_____

Length of Interview (hh:mm):_____

Interview Location:_____

Interviewer Name:___ _____

Cultural Beliefs and Intergenerational Relationships among Culturally Diverse Adults Interview Guide

SECTION A – INTRODUCTION AND INFORMED CONSENT

Hi [name of participant] and thank you for your time today. I'm [name of research] and I'm a [research assistant/graduate student researcher] at UC Berkeley. Before we begin, I first need to go over the consent form with you.

[*RESEARCHER: Reference the consent form and obtain either in-person or verbal consent over the phone. Sign and date the consent form indicating that you have gone through the consent form and the participant voluntarily agrees to participate.*]

Do you have any questions about the study before we begin? [If yes, answer questions.]

First, I would like to ask you to complete a survey. After that, I will ask you additional questions about your family's cultural background and beliefs, including yourself, one of your children, and one of your parents.

[*Researcher: Assist the participant with completing the survey. Once the survey is completed, continue with the interview.*]

SECTION B – CULTURAL IDENTITY AND RELATIONSHIP WITH THE AMERICAN BORN CHILD

Next, I would like to ask you a few questions about the [Japanese/Chinese/Hispanic] cultural beliefs and values of one of your children who was born in the Unites States and your relationship with this child.

1. Without mentioning a name, please let me know the current age and gender of this child.

(Please specify: Age: Sex:)

2. In your opinion, how does your child view his/her [Japanese/Chinese/Hispanic] cultural background and values?

3. In your opinion, how does your child view American culture in the U.S?

Next, I would like to ask you a few questions about your perspectives of parental support for this child.

4. What kind of parental support do you believe your child expects from you, if any?
[PROMPT: For example, supports may include emotional support, financial support, completion of household chores, helping him/her find information, and taking care of him/her when he/she is sick].
[PROBE: How much parental support do you believe your child expects from you?]

5. What kind of parental support do you believe you should provide for your child, if any?
[PROMPT: For example, supports may include emotional support, financial support, completion of household chores, helping him/her find information, and taking care of him/her when he/she is sick]
[PROBE: How much parental support do you believe you should provide to your child?]

Next, think about your relationship with this child,

6. How would you describe your relationship with this child?
[PROBE: How close do you feel you are to your child?]
[PROBE: What kinds of conflicts do you have with your child?]

SECTION C – CULTURAL IDENTITY AND RELATIONSHIP WITH THE PARENT

Now, we would like to ask you a few questions about the [JAPANESE/CHINESE/HISPANIC] cultural beliefs and values of one of your parents and your relationship with this parent.

7. Without mentioning a name, please tell me the current age and gender of this parent.
(Please specify: Age: Sex:)

Appendix   185

8. In your opinion, how does your parent view his/her [JAPANESE/CHINESE/ HISPANIC] cultural background and values?

9. In your opinion, how does your parent view American culture?

Next, I would like to ask you a few questions about your perspectives of family support for this parent.

10. What kind of family support do you believe your parent expects from you, if any?
[PROMPT: For example, supports may include emotional and physical support, financial support, completion of household chores, helping him/her find information, and taking care of him/her when he/she is sick].
[PROBE: How much family support do you believe your parent expects from you?]

11. What kind of family support do you believe you should provide for your parent, if any?
[PROMPT: For example, supports may include emotional and physical support, financial support, completion of household chores, helping him/her find information, and taking care of him/her when he/she is sick]
[PROBE: How much family support do you believe you should provide to your parent?]

Next, think about your relationship with this parent.

12. How would you describe your relationship with this parent?
[PROBE: How close do you feel you are to your parent?]
[PROBE: What kinds of conflicts do you have with your parent?]

SECTION D – CULTURAL IDENTITY AND FAMILY RELATIONSHIP AND SUPPORT

We are almost finished. Next, I would like to ask you a few questions about your [JAPANESE/CHINESE/HISPANIC] cultural beliefs and values and how they shape your relationships and expectations of your family members.

13. How do you view your [JAPANESE/CHINESE/HISPANIC] cultural background and values?

14. How do you view American culture?

Next, I would like to ask you a few questions about your perspectives of family support from your children.

186

15. What kind of family support do you believe your children feel they should provide for you, if any?

[PROMPT: For example, supports may include emotional support, financial support, completion of household chores, helping you find information, and taking care of you when you are sick].

[PROBE: How much family support do you believe your children feel they should provide for you?]

16. What kind of family support do you believe your children should provide for you if any?

[PROMPT: For example, supports may include emotional support, financial support, completion of household chores, helping you find information, and taking care of you when you are sick]

[PROBE: How much family support do you believe your children should provide for you?]

Next, I would like to ask you a few questions about family support from your parents.

17. What kind of family support do you believe your parents feel they should provide for you, if any?

[PROMPT: For example, supports may include emotional support, financial support, completion of household chores, helping you find information, and taking care of you when you are sick].

[PROBE: How much family support do you believe your parents feel they should provide for you?]

18. What kind of family support do you believe your parents should provide for you if any?

[PROMPT: For example, supports may include emotional support, financial support, completion of household chores, helping you find information, and taking care of you when you are sick]

[PROBE: How much family support do you believe your parents should provide to you?]

SECTION E – CONDCLUDING THE INTERVIEW

19. Finally, is there anything else that you would like to share with me about family support and your relationships with your child and parent?

Thank you so much for your time today. It is very much appreciated.

Appendix 4

The Multigroup Ethnic Identity Measure-Revised (Chapter 4)

Use the numbers given below to indicate how much you agree or disagree with each statement.

		1 Strongly disagree	2 Somewhat disagree	3 Moderate	4 Somewhat Agree	5 Strongly agree
1	I have spent time trying to find out more about my ethnic group, such as its history, traditions, and customs.	1	2	3	4	5
2	I have a strong sense of belonging to my own ethnic group.	1	2	3	4	5
3	I understand pretty well what my ethnic group membership means to me.	1	2	3	4	5
4	I have often done things that will help me understand my ethnic background better.	1	2	3	4	5
5	I have often talked to other people in order to learn more about my ethnic group.	1	2	3	4	5
6	I have a strong attachment towards my own ethnic group.	1	2	3	4	5

Appendix 5

The Multigroup Ethnic Identity Measure-Revised Japanese Version (Chapter 4)

あなた自身についてお聞きします。それぞれの文章が、あなたにどのくらいあてはまるかについて考えて、いちばんよくあてはまる番号にマル印をつけてください。

		1 まったくあてはまらない	2 ほとんどあてはまらない	3 あまりあてはまらない	4 かなりあてはまる	5 とてもよくあてはまる
1	私は、これまでに日本人のこと（歴史、文化、慣習など）をより深く知ろうとしてきた。	1	2	3	4	5
2	私は、自分が日本人であることを強く意識する。	1	2	3	4	5
3	私は、自分が日本人であることが、どのような意味をもつか、よく理解している。	1	2	3	4	5
4	私は、自分の日本人としての文化的背景について、よりよく理解するようなことをしてきた。	1	2	3	4	5
5	私は、しばしば、日本人のことをより深く知るために、他の人と話し合ってきた。	1	2	3	4	5
6	私は、日本人に強い愛着を感じる。	1	2	3	4	5

Contributor Biographies

Editor

Kazumi Hoshino is a Visiting Professor at the Osaka School of International Public Policy at Osaka University in Japan. She was a Residential Faculty Fellow at the Institute of East Asian Studies at the University of California at Berkeley (2011-2012). Dr. Hoshino was also appointed as a Visiting Scholar at the School of Public Health (2010-2011) and at the Institute of Personality and Social Research, (2012-2013) at the University of California at Berkeley as well as in the Department of Human Development and Family Studies at the Pennsylvania State University (2006-2007, 2013-2014). Dr. Hoshino's research interests include international migration, transdisciplinary and multicultural support for diverse immigrants, health policies, as well as healthy aging in the United States, Sweden, and Japan. She is a co-editor of the book, *Healthy Aging in Sociocultural Context.* New York: Routledge (2012), and a co-translator-in-chief of the Japanese book, *Healthy Aging in Sociocultural Context Japanese Version [Kenko Chojyu no Shakai Bunkateki Bunmyaku].* Tokyo: Kazamashobo Press (2013).

Co-Authors

Dolores Gallagher-Thompson is a Professor (Research) in the Department of Psychiatry and behavioral Science at the School of Medicine at Stanford University and a Director of the Outreach, Recruitment, and Education Core at the Alzheimer's Disease Research Center at Stanford University. Dr. Gallagher-Thompson was also a Director at the Stanford Geriatric Education Center at Stanford University. Her research has focused psychoeducational programs for family caregivers, impact on diversity on mental health, designing and implementing technology for mental health concerns, and cognitive/behavioral therapy for late life depression. Dr. Gallagher-Thompson recently published two books: *Geriatric Psychiatry: Cognitive Behavioral Therapy with Older Adults. In Comprehensive Textbook of Psychiatry* (B. J. Sadock & V. A. Sadock, Editors) (2016); and *Entries on CBT and Aging, and CBT and Caregiving, In International Encyclopedia of Cognitive Behavior Therapy* (A. Freeman, Editor) (2016).

Nancy Hikoyeda is retired from the Stanford Geriatric Education Center where she served as the Associate Director and Coordinator of the Faculty Development Program in Ethnogeriatrics. She was previously the Director of the Gerontology Program at San Jose State University and past president of the California Council on Gerontology and Geriatrics. Dr. Hikoyeda's areas of expertise include Asian/Pacific Islander elders, health literacy, cultural humility/cultural competence, and end-of-life issues. She has co-authored and edited numerous curriculum and training materials as well as book chapters on Asian American elders and their families. She is a co-author of the monograph, *Patient Listening: Health Communication Needs of Older Immigrants,* Philadelphia: Center for Intergenerational Learning, Temple University (2006), and a chapter entitled *Ethnic and Cultural Considerations in Care Management. In the Handbook of Geriatric Care Management* (C.J. Cress, Editor), Santa Cruz: Jones & Bartlett Learning (2015).

Winston Tseng is a Research Scientist and Lecturer in the Division of Community Health and Human Development at the School of Public Health and in the Department of Ethnic Studies at the University of California at Berkeley. Dr. Tseng is a medical sociologist with 20 years of participatory design and research experiences and partnerships with diverse, vulnerable populations, particularly Asian ethnic communities and the community-based organizations (CBOs) that serve them in California and across the United States. Dr. Tseng received his B.A. in Biology at Johns Hopkins University and his Ph.D. in Sociology at the University of California at San Francisco. Dr. Tseng's select publications include: Tseng, W., Huang, P., & Cook, W.C. (2011). Reshaping Data and Research through the Affordable Care Act: Opportunities for Asian American, Native Hawaiian and Pacific Islander Health. *AAPI Nexus, 9*(1), 193-204; and *Healthy Aging for Diverse Older Adults in the United States. In Healthy Aging in Sociocultural Context* (A. E. Scharlach & K. Hoshino, Editors), New York: Routledge (2012).

International Migration and Wellness Innovation
in the United States, Sweden, and Japan

2017年2月10日　初版第1刷発行

編著者　　星　野　和　実

発行者　　風　間　敬　子

発行所　　株式会社風間書房
〒101-0051　東京都千代田区神田神保町 1-34
電話 03(3291)5729　FAX 03(3291)5757
振替 00110-5-1853

印刷　太平印刷社　　製本　井上製本所

©2017　　　　　　　　　　　　　NDC 分類：140
ISBN978-4-7599-2173-1　　Printed in Japan

JCOPY 〈(社)出版者著作権管理機構　委託出版物〉

本書の無断複製は，著作権法上での例外を除き禁じられています。複製される
場合はそのつど事前に(社)出版者著作権管理機構（電話 03-3513-6969，FAX 03-
3513-6979，e-mail: info@jcopy.or.jp）の許諾を得て下さい。